Current Themes in Psychiatry in Theory and Practice

Current Themes in Psychiatry in Theory and Practice

Edited by

Niruj Agrawal
St George's Hospital, London, UK

Jim Bolton
St Helier Hospital, Carshalton, UK

and

Raghunandan Gaind
Keats House, London, UK

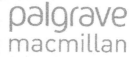

First published 2012 by
PALGRAVE MACMILLAN

Palgrave Macmillan in the UK is an imprint of Macmillan Publishers Limited, registered in England, company number 785998, of Houndmills, Basingstoke, Hampshire RG21 6XS.

Palgrave Macmillan in the US is a division of St Martin's Press LLC, 175 Fifth Avenue, New York, NY 10010.

Palgrave Macmillan is the global academic imprint of the above companies and has companies and representatives throughout the world.

Palgrave® and Macmillan® are registered trademarks in the United States, the United Kingdom, Europe and other countries.

ISBN 978-1-349-35827-4   ISBN 978-0-230-31706-2 (eBook)
DOI 10.1057/9780230317062

This book is printed on paper suitable for recycling and made from fully managed and sustained forest sources. Logging, pulping and manufacturing processes are expected to conform to the environmental regulations of the country of origin.

A catalogue record for this book is available from the British Library.

Library of Congress Cataloging-in-Publication Data

Current themes in psychiatry in theory and practice / edited by Niruj Agrawal, Jim Bolton, Raghunandan Gaind.
      p. ; cm.
   Includes bibliographical references and index.

   1. Psychiatry. 2. Mental illness. I. Agrawal, Niruj. II. Bolton, Jim, 1965– III. Gaind, Raghunandan [DNLM: 1. Psychiatry. 2. Mental Disorders. WM 100]
RC454.C826 2011
616.89—dc23   2011013735

The Practice of medicine is an art not trade, a calling, not a business. A calling in which your heart will be exercised equally with your head.

Sir William Osler, 1903

Contents

Part I   Issues of Contemporary Concern

Part II   Interface of Medicine and Psychiatry

Part III Therapeutic Challenges

Tables

Figures

Boxes

Abbreviations

ABGA	anti-basal ganglia antibodies
ACE	Addenbrooke's Cognitive Examination
ACTH	adrenocorticotrophic hormone
ADHD	attention deficit hyperactivity disorder
ADR	acute dystonic reaction
ADRDA	Alzheimer's Disease and Related Disorders Association
AIDS	acquired immune deficiency syndrome
AIREN	Association Internationale pour la Recherche et l'Enseignment en Neurosciences
ANS	autonomic nervous system
ASD	autistic spectrum disorder
ATPD	acute and transient psychotic disorder
BAD	bipolar affective disorder
BDI	Beck Depression Inventory
BMI	body mass index
BPD	borderline personality disorder
BSE	bovine spongiform encephalopathy
CADASIL	cerebral autosomal dominant arteriopathy with subcortical infarcts and leukoencephalography
CBT	cognitive-behavioural therapy
CD	conduct disorder
CI	confidence interval
CJD	Creutzfeldt–Jakob disease
CMT	chronic motor or vocal tic disorder
CNS	central nervous system
COMPASS	Combined Psychosis and Substance Use Programme
COPD	chronic obstructive pulmonary disease
CREATE	Cardiac Randomized Evaluation of Antidepressant and Psychotherapy Efficacy
CSF	cerebrospinal fluid
CSM	Committee on Safety of Medicines
CT	computed tomography
CYP	cytochrome P450
DAT-SPECT	dopamine transporter single proton emission computed tomography

DBS	deep brain stimulation
DBT	dialectical behaviour therapy
DEXA	dual x-ray absorptiometry
DOP	dangerous offender provisions
DOSMED	Determinants of Outcome of Serious Mental Disorders Study
DSM	*Diagnostic and Statistical Manual of Mental Diseases*
DSPD	Dangerous and Severe Personality Disorder (initiative)
ECG	electrocardiography/electrocardiographic
ECT	electroconvulsive therapy
EDNOS	eating disorders not otherwise specified
EEG	electroencephalogram/electroencephalography
EMG	electromyogram/electromyography
EOG	electro-oculography
ENRICHD	Enhancing Recovery in Coronary Heart Disease (trial)
EPS	extrapyramidal symptoms
ESR	erythrocyte sedimentation rate
FBC	full blood count
FLAIR	fluid attenuated inversion recovery
fMRI	functional magnetic resonance imaging
FNEA	functional non-epileptic attacks
FTD	frontotemporal dementia
GABA	gamma amino butyric acid
GABHS	group A beta-haemolytic streptococcus
GHQ	General Health Questionnaire
GSR	galvanic skin response
HAART	highly active antiretroviral therapy
HCR-20	Historical Clinical Risk-20
5-HIAA	5-hydroxyindole acetic acid
HIV	human immunodeficiency virus
HMPAO	hexamethylpropyleneamine oxime
HRT	habit-reversal training
HRV	heart-rate variability
ICD	*International Classification of Diseases*
IHCIS	Integrated Healthcare Information Services
IPD	idiopathic Parkinson's disease
IPP	Indeterminate Public Protection (order)
IPSS	International Pilot Study of Schizophrenia
IR	International Registry
ITU	intensive therapy unit
LFT	liver function test

LIT	local implementation team
LSP	language-support programme
MAO$_A$	monoamine oxidase A
MBT	mentalisation-based therapy
MET	motivational enhancement therapy
MMPI	Minnesota Multiphasic Personality Inventory
MMSE	mini mental state examination
MND	motor neurone disease
MRI	magnetic resonance imaging
NA	Narcotics Anonymous
NCS-R	National Comorbidity Survey replication
NEAD	non-epileptic attack disorder
NHS	National Health Service
NHSDA	National Household Survey on Drug Abuse
NICE	National Institute for Health and Clinical Excellence
NINCDS	National Institute of Neurological and Communication Disorders and Stroke
NINDS	National Institute of Neurological Disorders and Stroke
NIP	neuroleptic-induced parkinsonism
NL	neuroleptic
NMDA	*N*-methyl-D-aspartate
NSF	National Service Framework
NSMHW	National Survey of Mental Health and Wellbeing
OCB	obsessive-compulsive behaviour
OCD	obsessive-compulsive disorder
OCP	oral contraceptive pill
ODD	oppositional defiant disorder
PANDAS	paediatric autoimmune neuropsychiatric disorders associated with streptococcal infections
PCL-R	revised version of the Psychotherapy Checklist
PD	personality disorder
PET	positron emission tomography
PHQ	Patient Health Questionnaire
PNES	psychogenic non-epileptic seizures
PTSD	post-traumatic stress disorder
QEEG	quantitative EEG
QOL	quality of life
QOLAS	Quality of Life Assessment Schedule
QTc	QT interval corrected for heart rate
RBD	rapid eye movement sleep behaviour disorder
RCT	randomised controlled trial

REM	rapid eye movement
RLS	restless legs syndrome
RSA	respiratory sinus arrhythmia
SADHART	Sertraline Antidepressant Heart Attack Randomized Trial
SAMHSA	Substance Abuse and Mental Health Services Administration
SCAAPS	Schedule for the Clinical Assessment of Acute Psychotic States
SFT	schema-focused therapy
SIB	self-injurious behaviour
SPECT	single proton emission computed tomography
SSRI	selective serotonin reuptake inhibitor
T_3	tri-iodothyronine
T_4	thyroxine
TCA	tricyclic antidepressant
TD	tardive dyskinesia
TFP	transference-focused psychotherapy
TFT	thyroid function test
TS	Tourette syndrome
TSH	thyroid-stimulating hormone
TTD	thought-translation device
UK	United Kingdom
USA	United States of America
UNESCO	United Nations Educational, Scientific and Cultural Organization
vCJD	new variant Creutzfeldt–Jakob disease
VRAG	Violence Risk Appraisal Guide
WHO	World Health Organization

Preface

Psychiatry as a discipline has been growing at an astounding rate internationally. There has been a rapid expansion of services to meet the needs of mentally ill people. In parallel, ongoing research has led to a dramatic explosion of information. It is a formidable task to keep up to date with knowledge and this is a great challenge for teachers and clinicians. *Current Themes in Psychiatry in Theory and Practice* strives to help trainees and busy clinicians keep abreast of issues of contemporary concern and therapeutic challenges in clinical psychiatry.

Current Themes in Psychiatry was published as a series of books from the late 1970s to the early 1990s under the leadership of its lead editor Dr Raghunandan Gaind. The book proved useful to psychiatrists preparing for higher examinations as well as to others in allied disciplines with special interest in psychiatry. Volumes 3 and 4 included more international contributions, particularly from North America, on varying topics reflecting the developments in modern psychiatry and examining new psychotherapies.

The core purpose of the current book is to provide a clinically relevant and detailed overview of carefully selected topics. These topics are often not covered in as much detail by commonly read textbooks and we hope this book will complement those textbooks. Busy clinicians and trainees may not have enough time to do their own detailed literature searches, or may not have access to the vast array of journal articles that inform various chapters of this book. We have chosen authors who are leaders in their fields and are experienced clinicians, researchers and writers. They have used their vast experience and clinical wisdom to distil the essential information from the published literature to date and present it in a manner that is easy to follow for the reader whilst instilling greater insights.

The book consists of 14 chapters covering a wide range of psychiatric topics divided into three sections. Part I focuses on issues of contemporary concern including chapters on highly topical and globally relevant areas such as 'Culture and Mental Health' and 'Public Health Psychiatry in Criminal Justice States'. In an increasingly shrinking and globalised world with constant and ongoing migration in all directions, conceptual knowledge and practical understanding of cultural issues is a must for all clinicians. The second chapter deals with the conflict that most psychiatrists face between duty to society and their duty to the individual. With an ageing society and increasing focus on dementia in the elderly, there is recognition of glaring gap in knowledge and service provision for younger people with dementia, which is covered in the third chapter. Chapters 4 and 5 provide a much needed reconsideration of the topics of 'Substance Misuse and Comorbid Psychiatric Disorders' and 'Acute and Transient Psychotic Disorders', which remain a source of diagnostic and management dilemma globally.

Part II deals with often-overlooked 'Interface of Medicine and Psychiatry'. Chapter 6 deals with 'Symptoms Unexplained by Disease', which is a subject everyone finds difficult, and clinically useful information is often difficult to come by. The chapter on 'Functional Non-epileptic Attacks' nicely complements the one on 'Symptoms Unexplained by Disease'. Chapters on 'Tourette Syndrome', 'Depression in Physical Illness' and 'Physical Consequences of Eating Disorders' highlight the extensive interface between medicine and psychiatry and provide readers with practical insights.

Part III focuses on therapeutic challenges and advances in contemporary psychiatry. Despite the emergence of a whole range of atypical antipsychotic drugs with promise of no extrapyramidal side effects, the topic of 'Neuroleptic-induced Movement Disorders' remains as relevant as ever. The challenge of helping patients to take medications as prescribed is felt by clinicians worldwide and is nowhere else more acute than in the area of antidepressant prescribing, as discussed in Chapter 12. Emerging treatments in two very different areas are discussed in the last two chapters: 'Borderline Personality Disorder' and 'Biofeedback in Psychiatric Practice', providing readers with an overview as well as necessary clinical understanding.

We believe this book will help in guiding psychiatry students worldwide. It will also be a useful resource for busy psychiatrists in day-to-day clinical practice, and for other medical and allied professionals such as general practitioners, psychologists, mental health nurses and social workers, to name a few. We hope the variety of chapters included will enhance and stimulate clinicians and lead to a better clinical care.

We are grateful for the encouragement and practical advice we have received throughout from Dr Raghunandan Gaind, founder of the original series to whom this book is dedicated. This book would not have been possible without the help and support of many people. We would like to thank all the authors for their outstanding contributions, which are both scholarly and easy to read. We have the pleasure of knowing them all and working with many of them. We are grateful to Olivia Middleton, Associate Editor at Palgrave Macmillan, for her support and friendly advice, and Rebecca Ewens for proof reading. Thank you to our families for their constant support during the editing and production of this book.

Niruj Agrawal and Jim Bolton

Foreword

I am delighted to have been asked to provide a foreword to *Current Themes in Psychiatry in Theory and Practice.*

It has been my good fortune to have had the benefit of previously attending lectures or reading papers by the majority of the authors, a distinguished group of British psychiatrists and neurologists. What makes this volume so welcome is that their relevant clinical experience is coupled with strong commitment to the rigours of science and evidence-based practice and healthy scepticism about fads of one sort or another. Though all are practising in the UK, the authoritative and up-to-date nature of their reviews and the special care that they have taken to make them accessible to the busy clinician make this collection of immediate practical relevance to international as well as British readers.

This is a collection of reviews fit to refine the practice of the experienced specialist as well as shape the practice and examinations preparation of the psychiatric trainee. The various authors have extensive clinical experience in the fields they review and this stands out immediately on first reading. For example, in my own field of liaison psychiatry, I found the chapter by Carson and Stone on 'Symptoms Unexplained by Disease' consistent with my practice but it also gave me new practical hints that would benefit my patients in the future. As well as the liaison psychiatrist, the general adult psychiatrist and other psychiatrists that come across somatising patients will benefit in practice from reading this chapter.

Psychiatry is a broad and evolving discipline. The present selection fairly, and in a balanced way, reflects the breadth of the discipline in adult clinical psychiatry, with chapters from a wide variety of fields, from transcultural psychiatry to neuropsychiatry, from psychosis to symptoms unexplained by disease, from substance misuse to eating disorders, from Tourette syndrome to borderline personality disorder, and so on. Some fear that psychiatry is under threat. This volume points to its strength.

George Ikkos BSC, LMSSA, FRCPsych, MInstGA
Consultant Psychiatrist in Liaison Psychiatry,
Royal National Orthopaedic Hospital
Hon. Visiting Research Professor, London South Bank University
Hon. Treasurer, Royal College of Psychiatrists

Editors

Niruj Agrawal is Consultant Neuropsychiatrist and Honorary Senior Lecturer at the Atkinson Morley Regional Neurosciences Centre London, UK. He is a member of the Royal College of Psychiatrists, British Neuropsychiatric Association, American Neuropsychiatric Association and International Neuropsychiatric Association. He is the Vice Chair of the Neuropsychiatry section of the Royal College of Psychiatrists. He is actively involved in teaching and has published several scientific papers, book chapters and has edited *The Blue Book* for his trust since 2003.

Jim Bolton is Consultant Liaison Psychiatrist at St Helier Hospital in London, and an Honorary Senior Lecturer at St George's University of London, UK. He has a particular interest in medical education. He is the Director of Medical Education for South West London and St George's Mental Health NHS Trust, has extensive experience in teaching undergraduate and postgraduate doctors in training, and also has an interest in educating the general public on mental health. He has published on a variety of aspects of mental illness, including liaison psychiatry, eating disorders and stigma.

Raghunandan Gaind is Consultant Neuropsychiatrist, Keats House, London, UK.

Contributors

Mohammed T. Abou-Saleh is Professor of Psychiatry and Honorary Consultant in Addiction Psychiatry, St George's, University of London, UK.

Dinesh Bhugra is Professor of Mental Health and Cultural Diversity, President of The Royal College of Psychiatrists, Institute of Psychiatry, London, UK.

Alan Carson is Consultant Neuropsychiatrist and Part Time Senior Lecturer, Department of Clinical Neurosciences, University of Edinburgh, Western General Hospital, Edinburgh, Scotland.

Kishore Chandiramani is Consultant Psychiatrist, Nuffield Health, North Staffordshire Hospital, Newcastle under Lyme, UK.

Sanjoo Chengappa is Academic Clinical Fellow, St George's University of London, UK.

Danielle Gaynor is Assistant Psychologist, East London Foundation Trust, UK.

Pat Hughes is Professor of Psychotherapy, Head of Division of Mental Health, St George's University of London, UK.

George Ikkos is Consultant Psychiatrist in Liaison Psychiatry, Royal National Orthopaedic Hospital, London, UK.

Kate Jefferies is Consultant Old Age Psychiatrist, Farnham Road Hospital, Guildford, Surrey, UK.

J. Hubert Lacey is Professor of Psychiatry and Clinical Director, St George's Eating Disorders Service, London, UK.

Robert Lawrence is Consultant Old Age Psychiatrist and Honorary Senior Lecturer, Barnes Hospital, London, UK.

Marie-Hélène Marion is Consultant Neurologist with the Movement Disorders Unit, Atkinson Morley Regional Neurosciences Centre, St George's Hospital, London, UK.

Alex J. Mitchell is Consultant and Honorary Senior Lecturer in Liaison Psychiatry, Leicester Royal Infirmary, Leicester, UK.

John Morgan is Consultant Psychiatrist in Eating Disorders, Yorkshire Centre for Eating Disorders, UK.

Audrey Ng is Specialist Registrar in Psychiatry, Department of Liaison Psychiatry, St Mary's Hospital, London, UK.

Norman Poole is Locum Consultant in Liaison Psychiatry, St Bartholomew's Hospital, London, UK.

Steven Reid is Consultant in Liaison Psychiatry, Department of Liaison Psychiatry, St Mary's Hospital, London, UK.

Daniel C. Riordan is Consultant Forensic Psychiatrist, Psychotherapist and Group Analyst, Justice Health, Sydney, Australia.

Mary M. Robertson is Professor and Honorary Consultant Neuropsychiatrist, Department of Mental Health Sciences, University College London, London, UK.

Jaydip Sarkar is Consultant Forensic Psychiatrist, Personality Disorder Unit and Secure Women's Services, East Midlands Centre for Forensic Mental Health, Leicester, UK.

Swaran P. Singh is Professor of Social and Community Psychiatry and Consultant Psychiatrist, Health Sciences Research Institute, University of Warwick, Coventry, UK.

Jeremy S. Stern is Consultant Neurologist, Atkinson Morley Regional Neurosciences Centre, St George's Hospital, London, UK.

Jon Stone is Consultant Neurologist and Honorary Senior Lecturer, Department of Clinical Neurosciences, University of Edinburgh, Western General Hospital, Edinburgh, UK.

Kate Webb is Specialist Registrar and Honorary Research Assistant, St George's Eating Disorders Service, London, UK.

Part I
Issues of Contemporary Concern

1
Culture and Mental Health

Dinesh Bhugra and Norman Poole

Culture, that which is cultivated, has traditionally been contrasted with nature, that which we are born into. Nature is universal, invariable and physically present. Tylor, an early anthropologist, conceived culture as '[the] complex whole which includes knowledge, beliefs, art, law, morals, custom and any other capabilities and habits acquired by man as a member of society'.[1] He held that each individual human had the same innate capacities but some societies had a more developed culture than others, with the less developed cultures gradually progressing to a more evolved state. While the theory of cultural evolution was soon jettisoned, Tylor's definition has been broadly retained by much of 20th-century anthropology. For example, a recent definition of culture was provided by Fitzgerald et al.: 'Culture is an abstract concept that refers to learned, shared patterns of perceiving and adapting to the world which is reflected in the learned, shared beliefs, values, attitudes and behaviours characteristic of a society or population'.[2] Culture thus provides normative standards of behaviour, regulating what a person ought and ought not to do in any given situation.

The culture that one belongs to existed before one's birth and will persist, with perhaps some minor changes, beyond one's death. And all the events that occur during a lifetime derive their meaning and value through culture. As the definitions above make clear, culture is that part of being human that is learned. The process begins from birth with the acts of naming, dressing and rearing in accordance with rules set down within the parents' culture and continues throughout the lifetime, being influenced by peers, educational system, society and through components of culture such as training, religion, language, media etc. The values and traditions that are transmitted from one generation to the next bind those who share them into a community, which in turn ensures the propagation of that culture.

Cultural identity refers to the sense individuals have of their own values, beliefs, attitudes, style of communication and patterns of behaviour – what cultural community they identify themselves with. However, this should not be taken to imply that culture is homogeneous and cultural identification stable. A person may identify with one or more subcultures within their culture, this can change over time and cultural identification can alter depending upon circumstance. So for example, a Muslim mental health professional may identify with her religious heritage at home, but at work the culture of mental health practice and caring comes to the fore. There are also subcultures with specific identity for female and Muslim psychiatrists, either of which she may or may not identify with. Religious and cultural rites of passage assist the formation of cultural identity, and the extent to which an individual is accepted by a community is influenced by his or her degree of conformity to the cultural rules and rituals.

Cultural identity should not be confused with social identity, though the two concepts are related.[3] Social identity is the culturally defined value and expectations that are ascribed to particular social roles, such as fatherhood, friendship, and particular occupational roles like that of the physician. Within the so-called bourgeois family in western society, the father was expected to provide financially and make crucial decisions but not to be directly involved in parenting, which was left to female family members. This changing social identity illustrates that different cultures value and expect different things from the same role and that these traditions are not immutable.

Ethnicity too is a related but not identical concept that has typically incorporated aspects of both race and culture. Individuals who constitute an ethnic group share a common heritage that can be religious, tribal, geographic, related to nationality, historical or physical. However, a key controversy is whether race is a biologically valid idea or whether it is a social construct that serves social purposes. The idea behind the race concept for the last hundred years or more has been a genetic and biological one as illustrated in this dictionary definition.

Race – large group of people with common ancestry and inherited physical characteristics. (*Oxford English Dictionary*)

The biologically based race concept fits people to a group defined by one or more of (a) shared physical characteristics, for example skin colour, facial features and hair texture, (b) geographical origins and (c) ancestral origins.

The idea that each 'race' has distinct biological characteristics that could be considered more or less valuable justified policies of discrimination, exclusion, forced sterilisation and even extermination throughout the 20th century. In the 1950s the United Nations Educational, Scientific and Cultural Organization (UNESCO) published *The Race Question*,[4] a document signed by many of the leading biological and social scientists of the day, which criticised the concept of race and advocated speaking instead of ethnicity. Thus conceived, ethnicity is more porous, dynamic and cultural than the biologically determined race concept. For example, people from the West Indies, Africa and parts of North and South America may share some physical features but have different beliefs, value systems and behavioural norms. Therefore, they constitute discrete ethnic groups.

Culture and psychiatry

The relationships between culture and psychiatry are manifold. In the first and most obvious sense, the mental health professions have their own unique training and mode of practice, giving them each a distinctive culture. And each psychiatric institution and subspeciality develops its own culture that is identified with, to varying degrees, by its members.

With the rise of the anti-psychiatry critique, culture came to be seen as problematic for psychiatry and psychiatric concepts. As we see in the next section, abnormal behaviour and mental states are shaped and delimited by the culture in which they occur. Standard psychopathological concepts are now seen by some to be a cultural consequence of enlightenment thought dominant in the west. Psychiatry, far from sitting atop the solid base of a universal psychopathology, is relative. This school of thought has been particularly powerful in psychosomatic medicine, which now considers medically unexplained symptoms to be 'idioms of distress': a socially sanctioned and understood means to communicate intrapsychic or interpersonal conflict.

There are many ways that psychopathology can be influenced by culture, as clearly articulated by Tseng:[5]

1. pathogenic effect (cultural influence on the formation of a disorder)
2. psychoselective effect (culture selecting certain coping patterns to deal with stress)

3. psychoplastic effect (culture modifying the clinical manifestation)
4. pathoelaborating effect (culture elaborating mental conditions into a unique nature)
5. psychofacilitating effect (culture promoting the frequency of occurrence)
6. psychoreactive effect (culture shaping folk responses to the clinical condition).

In the sections we review the pathogenetic nature of acculturation, finding oneself in an alien culture, and cultural bereavement, before appraising some strategies to ameliorate this effect. The chapter ends with a review of cultural competence, and how it can be enhanced in the field of mental health.

Jaspers' model of form and content

As detailed at length in his *General Psychopathology*, Karl Jaspers identified that psychiatry's subject matter straddled both nature and culture:

> Although man *inherits* his bodily and psychic dispositions his actual psychic life is achieved only through *tradition* which reaches him through the human society that surrounds him.[6]

The admixture of nature and culture was significant in shaping his vision of psychopathology, which, it is well known, was based on differentiating form and content. The form of a psychopathological feature was determined by nature and so was universal among human beings. Content, on the other hand, was supplied by culture and so could be expected to vary between places and at different times. It would be wrong to conclude from this that Jaspers is suggesting that content is unimportant and can safely be ignored. Indeed, much of Jaspers' book is given over to investigating the so-called 'meaningful connections' that constitute content, and he is at pains to point out that 'it is by no means easy to define the borders between heredity and tradition in matters of psychic life'.[6]

Not all psychiatrists have been so circumspect with regard to this distinction, however. Kraepelin's application of psychopathological constructs derived from studies in western populations to the people of Java has been criticised by Littlewood as naïve.[7] Kraepelin, he argues, makes an assumption that some features of psychosis represent the true biological core of the disease, and so will be present in all cases, irrespective of ethnicity and culture. Differences in presentation that are discovered between cultures can then be regarded merely as colourful distractions. Kleinman makes the same complaint about the World Health Organization's (WHO's) International Pilot Study of Schizophrenia (IPSS),[8] which concludes that psychosis occurs with roughly the same frequency and pattern of symptoms in all countries and cultures. By focusing on a range of core features that are assumed to be biologically determined, the differences in the pattern of symptoms and their meaning to the person and his or her community are systematically ignored.

To consider psychopathological concepts as universally applicable has been called the 'etic' approach. So, for example, koro – the fear the penis is being retracted into the body, which will ultimately result in death – should not be regarded as an unusual and bizarre culturally dependent syndrome found exclusively in Asia. Instead, it is argued, this syndrome occurs only in those who adhere to the local belief that a fox spirit wants to remove their penis, which causes them to experience panic attacks and catastrophising cognitions and seek desperate measures within the family to prevent it from happening. Culture supplies the belief and illness behaviour but paroxysmal anxiety has a universal form.[9]

This can be contrasted with the 'emic' approach, which views the western model of psychopathology as culturally dependent, just like any other indigenous system. For example, Yap has proposed that Jaspers' distinction between form and content is only possible in Indo-European languages because these have a subject/predicate grammar.[10] Proponents of this school contend that symptom checklists can be reliably administered around the world but if the cultural meaning and social response of these symptoms are ignored, then the diagnostic categories generated are invalid.[8] Rather, symptoms should be construed as idioms of distress – behavioural phenomena that are meaningfully related to particular psychosocial stressors, communicate conflict and distress, and thereby elicit a caring response from their community.

Idioms of distress

Kleinman's work on neurasthenia in China is the exemplary illustration of this approach to psychiatry.[8] He found depression to be rare in China, in contrast to neurasthenia, which involves many of the somatic symptoms found in depression, such as weakness, fatigue, poor sleep and reduced appetite. Also, 87% of those diagnosed with neurasthenia responded well to tricyclic antidepressants. He suggests that expressions of low mood were poorly tolerated during the Maoist revolution and psychiatrists deemed politically reactionary, so interpersonal and intra-psychic conflicts were conveyed to and understood by others through the somatic symptoms. In America, a culture that encourages expression of distress though talking about psychological and emotional states, communication of distress through physical symptoms is taken to signify unusually poor coping resources. So the same set of symptoms in different cultures conveys different meanings and requires a quite different response.

The tendency for distress to be made manifest by physical symptoms is not restricted to China. Japanese students in Japan, in comparison with their American counterparts, report higher levels of somatic symptoms when depressed.[11] The particular symptoms experienced during a depressive episode also appear to vary across cultures. The Japanese complain more of headaches, skin changes, weakness and shoulder pain, which are generally omitted from western psychiatric assessment tools. These symptoms also symbolically convey information about that patient's world. Subtle alterations in somatic functioning signify social disharmony, in keeping with traditional Japanese concepts about balance and order. Indeed, the separation of symptoms into psychological and somatic is likely to be an artefact of western dualism (which predates Descartes by a couple of millennia) that has little validity in cultures that lack this dichotomy.

It would be an oversimplification and misrepresentation of the cultural psychiatrist's critique to suggest that all psychiatric symptoms, and therefore all psychiatric diagnoses, are culturally relative. Rather, each symptom should be taken as existing somewhere along a continuum between a fully biomedical explanation (such as the psychic manifestations of partial seizures) and at the other extreme a fully sociological one (shop-lifting, overdose, binging and purging). Most symptoms relevant to psychiatry will lie somewhere between these two poles and a hybrid biosocial model is required to provide a complete account of their origin and significance. It is noteworthy that Littlewood considers both modern cognitive psychology and psychoanalysis to be variations of folk psychology.[7] All cultures have implicit explanatory models used by the 'folk' to predict and explain their own and their fellows' behaviour. The particular folk psychological theory in use will therefore be interpreted from the anthropological perspective, or, to put it another way, from the social component of the biosocial model.

All these issues have significant practical relevance. As Bhui et al. note,[12] any survey of non-western populations that uses instruments not grounded by relevant ethnographic work is liable to give erroneous rates of mental illness in that community. Individual cases will be missed or mental disorder wrongly diagnosed and the provision of services will not be planned in accordance with local need.

Acculturation and cultural bereavement

Culture does not merely provide the rules dictating how distress should be displayed and managed; it can also be a source of that distress. People migrate to countries with unfamiliar cultures for a variety of reasons and purposes: to join friends or family, improve employment or educational opportunities, and to avoid political and religious persecution or avoid war and other catastrophes. In the United Kingdom (UK), the proportion of the population composed of non-white groups increased from 5.5% in 1991 to 7.9% by 2001. Ongoing conflicts and the likelihood of increased competition for resources as a consequence of climate change are unlikely to moderate this trend. Declining birth rates among indigenous whites in the west are contributing to a demographic shift that will be unsustainable without inward migration of workers. Societies, certainly in the west, are becoming increasingly plural whether they wish to or not. Migration is known to have a deleterious effect on some migrants

The changes that occur when two or more cultures come into sustained contact with one another is known as *acculturation*. Originally viewed exclusively from the perspective of the non-dominant culture, it is now acknowledged that each culture is modified in the process. Berry describes how acculturation operates at the level of the group (cultural acculturation) and individual (psychological acculturation), and how this impacts on mental health.[13] If a minority culture retains much of its heritage and traditions but engages with members from the dominant group, then it is said to be adopting a strategy of *integration*. *Assimilation* occurs when engagement is pursued and cultural identity is shed in favour of the dominant one. A low level of engagement, with retention of cultural traditions, results in *separation*, whereas loss of cultural identity but little engagement causes *marginalisation*. These strategies may be adopted by the group and individuals within the group. There will of course be significant variability in the extent individual members participate in the group strategy, which is influenced, among others things, by individual psychology. The potential for assimilation or integration strategies to be pursued depends upon the openness of the dominant culture. That is, does that culture value diversity and eschew racism and prejudice against the non-dominant cultural group.

Berry has conceptualised three types of outcome of acculturation. The first, unproblematic adaptation is called 'behavioural shifts' and involves three subprocesses: shedding patterns of behaviour inappropriate in the host culture; adopting new behaviours; and cultural conflict. Conflict occurs when the behaviour deemed inappropriate retains a high cultural value. It can be resolved by relinquishing to the dominant culture (assimilation), withdrawing into the original culture (separation), or agreeing a mutual accommodation (integration).

The second outcome type, 'acculturation stress', occurs when the level of cultural conflict is high but manageable and it is regarded as a chronic stressor. Integration is the strategy that causes the least stress, perhaps because it requires relatively little behavioural and psychological change from the group and its members. Some patterns of behaviour are gradually unlearned and replaced by those in keeping with the host culture but the greater part of cultural identity is maintained. Marginalisation, on the other hand, is the strategy associated with the highest levels of stress and psychopathology. Traditional support structures are undermined by the loss of cultural identity, which exclusion and rejection by the host culture exacerbates. Communities that have undergone marginalisation display high rates of delinquency, drug abuse and family breakdown. Unsurprisingly, migrants who have been pushed from their land of origin, such as refugees from war, report greater difficulties adapting than those who are positively drawn to the host country.

Severe acculturation difficulties have been called cultural bereavement by Eisenbruch, which he defines as:

> the experience of the uprooted person – or group – resulting from loss of social structures, cultural values and self-identity: the person – or group – continues to live in the past, is visited by supernatural forces from the past while asleep or awake, suffers feelings of guilt over abandoning culture and homeland, feels pain if memories of the past begin to fade, but finds constant images of the past (including traumatic images) intruding into daily life, yearns to complete obligations to the dead, and feels stricken by anxieties, morbid thoughts, and anger that mar the ability to get on with daily life.[14]

In young Cambodian war refugees who emigrated to Australia or the United States of America (USA), he found prolonged auditory and visual hallucinatory experiences involving ancestral spirits, particularly in those fostered into western families rather than Cambodian group homes. When the pattern of symptoms came to be assessed by psychiatrists they could receive a diagnosis of post-traumatic stress disorder or psychotic depression and be treated with medications. Eisenbruch however, recommends these experiences should be interpreted as cultural loss, and treatment should address this through reintegration with cultural and religious rituals and meaning. Medicalisation will, in fact, distance the individual from their cultural identity, with resultant further loss of self-esteem. So instead, Eisenbruch enabled the affected youths to meet with Buddhist monks and participate in *pcum-ben*, the annual ceremony held to venerate the dead.

Again, the issue is not that culturally dependent variability in the expression of psychological distress fatally undermines all psychiatric diagnosing; it is merely that culture significantly impacts how these experiences should be interpreted in each case. Psychiatric diagnoses cannot be applied without regard for the cultural context. Unfortunately, the current diagnostic systems (*International Classification of Diseases* [10th revised edition; ICD-10] and the *Diagnostic and Statistical Manual of Mental Diseases* [4th edition; DSM-IV]) retard the ability of clinicians to achieve this aim.

Evidence is beginning to accumulate that a strategy of integration causes the least mental disorder and distress, so indigenous mental health professionals should naturally advocate for a society that accepts and understands cultural difference. This approach, though, is far from ubiquitous in these professions themselves. However, the development of cultural competency is increasingly seen as an important attribute for psychiatrists and allied professionals.

Cultural competency

Patients from minority cultures are more likely to disengage from treatment and services, less likely to receive psychological interventions and so, unsurprisingly, report higher rates of dissatisfaction with their care. This has driven some to develop services with greater acceptance to minority groups, a broad strategy known as cultural competency. Cultural competency has been defined as: 'The ability of individuals to see beyond the boundaries of their own cultural interpretations, to be able to maintain objectivity when faced with individuals from cultures different from their own and be able to interpret and understand behaviours and intentions of people from other cultures non-judgementally and without bias'.[15] It is a capacity that has developed to varying degrees in individuals and organisations. To be culturally competent requires a broad range of skills and attributes such as cultural sensitivity, cultural knowledge, cultural empathy and self-awareness.[5, 16]

Cultural sensitivity is the recognition and respect for diversity of values, practices and beliefs, a willingness to learn more about cultures other than one's own and the avoidance of cultural stereotyping. Sensitivity, however, requires a degree of *cultural knowledge* – what are the rituals, customs, value systems and idioms of distress particular to the culture in question. Empathy is an essential requirement for any mental health professional but *cultural empathy* is the ability to enter into the patient's emotional experience despite any cultural differences that exist. These attributes can only be fostered in those with a degree of *self-awareness* for their attitudes to other cultural groups and appreciation that their own values and beliefs are largely culturally determined.

The culturally competent clinician is able to operate *effectively* in different cultural contexts for the benefit of patients. For example, cultural knowledge and sensitivity are required for the correct assessment of an Indian male who presents complaining of semen loss. The folk belief that 40 drops of food are required in the formation of one drop of blood and so on through flesh and marrow until finally semen is created is common in those from the Indian subcontinent.[17] This complaint thus frequently refers to fatigue and moral failure and is accompanied by foreboding and doom. If the clinician is unaware of this significance, then premature reassurance or an erroneous diagnosis of hypochondriacal disorder may be the outcome. Any proposed treatment is unlikely to be acceptable to a patient whose model of illness is at such variance with his clinician's.

The culturally competent mental health professional will also be aware of the structure of the doctor–patient relationship and how this impacts upon the consultation. This can prove a challenge when in conflict with the professional's own cultural values. Autonomy and confidentiality are now enshrined in medical practice in the west but in some cultures it is expected that family members will be told of the diagnosis and involved in decisions about treatment. In other instances, the patient's and clinician's cultural groups may have been in recent or traditional conflict, which produces a cultural transference and counter-transference that must be identified and managed.[18]

Level of cultural competence

Cross has proposed that an individual's or organisation's cultural competency lies somewhere on a continuum ranging from cultural destructiveness through cultural incapacity, cultural blindness, cultural pre-competence, to cultural competency, and finally cultural proficiency.[19] Further, he suggests that the majority of healthcare services operate around the cultural blindness to pre-competence range. Culturally blind organisations believe they deliver unbiased care but are in fact unreflectively ethnocentric. They apply their concepts of health and illness universally; assume all groups are the same; ignore cultural differences and strengths; and measure outcome solely against the mores and values of the dominant culture. Primacy is given to governmental policies that promote assimilation, though as Berry has shown, integration causes fewer acculturation difficulties and better mental health.[13] As services develop understanding of difference and a desire to deliver more culturally appropriate interventions, they enter the level of pre-competence. However, there is a danger of tokenism or false sense of accomplishment.

Services should always be aiming for cultural proficiency. Organisations at this stage value cultural difference and are continually expanding their knowledge base and developing culturally acceptable treatments. They employ culturally proficient staff and advocate for cultural competence in other agencies. Obviously from the descriptions given above, cultural competence is a process rather than a state, and organisations must continually monitor and refine their performance.

Improving cultural competence

Clinicians wishing to develop cultural competency must first establish where along the continuum their competence currently lies by asking themselves some awkward questions.

'Do I know how grief and distress are manifest in people from culture X?'

'Are there some features of this presentation that surprise and confuse me?'

'Do I assume certain facts about someone based on his or her culture?'

'Am I able to acknowledge and manage cultural transference and counter-transference?'

'If there is a gap in my knowledge, who do I approach to remedy this?'

'In cases of uncertainty, who do I approach to help resolve it?'

'Do my management plans include culturally appropriate strategies?'

'Do I explicitly acknowledge cultural differences with my patient?'
'Do I assess for cultural conflicts in my patients?'
'Am I someone who prefers cultural assimilation or integration?'

Individual cultural competence can be developed through specific programmes of education and training to increase cultural awareness and knowledge.[20] Lectures are cost-effective and convey large amounts of information about illness beliefs and idioms of distress but may not develop the requisite assessment skills and self-awareness. Case discussions draw out complexity and multiple perspectives while challenging attitudes and assumptions but, like role-play, do not increase participants' factual knowledge substantially. Given the growing importance of cultural competency in medical and psychiatric education, it is surprising that, as Bhui et al. point out, the method of teaching it has received so little evaluation. It is likely though that a combination of teaching methods with regular refresher courses is required if cultural proficiency is to be maintained.

However, culturally competent care can only be delivered if the entire organisation fosters respect and knowledge of diverse value systems, beliefs and practices. This can involve policies to ensure the ethnic make-up of the staff group mirrors the diversity found in the community being served. This is a contentious issue as it may encourage positive discrimination yet fail to provide the desired competency. Just because a person is of the same ethnic background, this is no guarantee they share a culture. Indeed, professional training immediately distances people's beliefs about illness, and other factors such as social class and religious grouping can create a further divide. Rather, it is better to put in place recruitment and retention policies that favour culturally competent clinicians from whatever background.

Basic training in cultural competency should be mandatory with more advanced programmes for those with an interest and aptitude to become local leaders, and a resource for others. Organisations may wish to facilitate a regular cultural consultation club, such as they have at St Bartholomew's Hospital in London, UK. These voluntary groups invite speakers to present research and complex cases and help to raise the profile and status of cultural psychiatry within the organisation.

A particularly interested clinician can immerse him or herself in another culture that is heavily represented in the catchment area through living-in working for a period in the country of origin, or becoming highly involved in the community. At any rate, links should be developed between the healthcare organisation and local community leaders and traditional healers. This is important because they are often approached with a problem long before the indigenous healthcare system. These links will enable efficient and culturally sanctioned referral to a mental healthcare professional where necessary, and in the other direction allows the clinician to instigate appropriate cultural support. Religious leaders can also be used when deciding whether a particular experience is culturally normal or shaded into psychopathology. For example, how many repetitions of the Rosary are required before the behaviour is deemed compulsive, and how long is it normal for Haitians to experience auditory hallucinations during a grief reaction? There should be ready access to interpreters trained in mental health assessment, which poses unique problems because of thought disorder, denial and the sometimes bizarre nature of experiences.

Kirmayer, et al. report on the development of their cultural consultation/liaison team.[21] Consultations took one of three forms. A consultant with requisite experience of the patient's culture provided an assessment over three sessions and then fed back a diagnosis and management plan directly to the referrer. Alternatively, the referrer and cultural consultant discussed the case and agreed a strategy but without directly assessing the patient. Finally, the cultural consultation team provided training and education to referring organisations, during which recurring difficulties and themes could be discussed and recommendations made. Almost all consultations (86%) were deemed beneficial by the referrer. Nearly half believed the consultation improved their treatment plan and one-third felt their understanding and therapeutic alliance had benefited.

Even if the organisation does not go so far as to develop a consultation/liaison team, they should be striving to make their services more acceptable to minority groups. A cultural competency plan should be drawn up at board level. This should include procedures to monitor the outcome and quality of care across differing ethnic groups and the development of an action plan if deficiencies are identified.

Conclusions

The actual value of cultural psychiatry continues to be debated. However, the extreme positions – that psychiatry and psychiatric diagnoses are rooted solely in culture and values with no biological reality whatsoever versus a pure biological reductionism – are no longer tenable.[22] The role played by culture will also vary from one condition to the next. Delirium probably appears similar in all cultures, though of course the content of delusions and hallucinations will differ, while more neurotic-type conditions will be considerably coloured by the sufferer's culture. The loss of culture, and cultural conflicts thrown up by migration, are detrimental to mental well-being. Given the increasing diversity of many countries, culture is an issue that will only become more prominent for clinicians, managers and researchers in the mental health field. Unfortunately, it remains true that many services play only lip service to cultural diversity and competence. There are strategies to improve these capacities in individual practitioners and the system in which they operate but, like all healthcare interventions, these need to be evaluated against desired outcomes. This is a pressing issue for the future.

Key learning points

● Culture influences how and where mental illness presents.
● Beliefs, values and behaviour are shaped by the agent's culture.
● Acculturation and cultural bereavement contribute to mental distress and disorder.
● Cultural competence enables effective health care across diverse cultures.
● Cultural competence can be fostered at the individual and organisational level.

References

1. Tylor E. *Primitive Culture*. New York: JP Putnam's Sons; 1920 [1871], p. 1.
2. Fitzgerald M, Mullavey-O'Byrne C, Clemson L. Cultural issues from practice. *Australian Occupational Therapy Journal* 1997; 44: 1–21.
3. Bhugra D, Becker MA. Migration, cultural bereavement and cultural identity. *World Psychiatry* 2004; 4(1): 18–24.
4. UNESCO. *The Race Question*. 1950.
5. Tseng W. From peculiar psychiatric disorders through culture-bound syndromes to culture-related specific syndromes. *Transcultural Psychiatry* 2006; 43: 554–76.
6. Jaspers K. *General Psychopathology*. Baltimore: John Hopkins University Press; 1997 [1959], p. 709.
7. Littlewood R. From categories to context: a decade of the 'new cross-cultural psychiatry'. *British Journal of Psychiatry* 1990; 156: 308–27.
8. Kleinman A. Anthropology and psychiatry: the role of culture in cross-cultural research on illness. *British Journal of Psychiatry* 1987; 151: 447–54.
9. Cheng A. Case definition and culture: are people all the same? *British Journal of Psychiatry* 2001; 179: 1–3.

10. Yap PM. *Comparative Psychiatry: a theoretical framework.* Toronto: University of Toronto Press; 1974.
11. Arnault DS, Sakamoto S, Moriwaki A. Somatic and depressive symptoms in female Japanese and American students: a preliminary investigation. *Transcultural Psychiatry* 2006; 43: 275–86.
12. Bhui K, Bhugra D, Goldberg D, Sauer J, Tylee A. Assessing the prevalence of depression in Punjabi and English primary care attenders: the role of culture, physical illness and somatic symptoms. *Transcultural Psychiatry* 2004; 41: 307–22.
13. Berry JW. Conceptual approaches to acculturation. In: Chun KM, Balls-Organista P Marín G, editors. *Acculturation: advances in theory, measurement, and applied research.* Washington, DC: American Psychological Association; 2003, pp. 17–37.
14. Eisenbruch M. From post-traumatic stress disorder to cultural bereavement: diagnosis of Southeast Asian refugees. *Social Science and Medicine* 1991; 33: 673–80.
15. Walker ML. *Rehabilitation Service Delivery to Individuals with Disabilities – A Question of Cultural Competence.* OSERS News in Print 1991; IV(2): 6
16. Adams DL. *Health Issues for Women of Color: a cultural diversity perspective.* Thousand Oaks: Sage Publications; 1995.
17. Sumathipala A, Siribaddana SH, Bhugra D. Culture-bound syndromes: the story of dhat syndrome. *British Journal of Psychiatry* 2004; 184: 200–209.
18. Comas-Díaz L, Jacobsen FM. Ethnocultural transference and countertransference in the therapeutic dyad. *American Journal of Orthopsychiatry* 1991; 61(3): 392–402.
19. Cross TL. *Towards a Culturally Competent System of Care: a monograph on effective services for minority children who are severely emotionally disturbed.* CASSP Technical Assistance Center; 2007 [1989].
20. Bhui K, Warfa N, Edonya P, McKenzie K, Bhugra D. Cultural competence in mental health care: a review of model evaluations. *BMC Health Services Research* 2007; 7: 15.
21. Kirmayer LJ, Groleau D, Guzder J, Blake C, Jarvis E. Cultural consultation: a model of mental health service for multicultural societies. *Canadian Journal of Psychiatry* 2003; 48(3): 145–53.
22. Bolton D. *What Is Mental Disorder: an essay in philosophy, science, and values.* Oxford: Oxford University Press; 2008.

2
Public Health Psychiatry in Criminal Justice States

Jaydip Sarkar

> There is nothing so shocking as madness in the cabin of the Irish peasant... When a strong man or woman gets the complaint, the only way they have to manage is by making a hole in the floor of the cabin, not high enough for the person to stand up in, with a crib over it to prevent his getting up. This hole is about five feet deep, and they give this wretched being his food there, and there he generally dies.
> (a member of the House of Commons, Irish District, 1817)

The statement above highlights the 'safety' aspect of the task of psychiatry – to keep the 'madman' safe from himself as well as from the European societies of mid-19th century with an authoritarian intolerance of, and increasingly brutal manners to gain control over, abnormal behaviour.[1] With the passage of time, the public health role, i.e. keeping societies safe from the 'madman', has become the public face of psychiatry. The profession has tried unsuccessfully to shed this image, and in recent times failed entirely in its attempts in face of severe societal and legislative pressures. It is suggested in this chapter that the (re)emergence of a predominant public health role of psychiatry lies embedded in the policies that many countries, most notably the United Kingdom (UK) and United States of America (USA), have been pursuing for some time now, such that these have become criminal justice states that nurture a culture of control.[2]

In recent times, with regard to managing the law and order situation, there has been a rapid dilution of penal welfarism, i.e. the notion that denial of liberties requires a reciprocal pursuit of rehabilitative ideals. This has occurred alongside a corresponding increase of punitive sanctions and just desserts retribution as a generalised policy goal.[2] These changes reversed the more liberal air that existed until three decades ago and have gathered momentum exponentially after recent global terrorist concerns. These concerns have elicited certain responses from state agencies, some of which are adaptive and others non-adaptive, and include amongst others, attempts to (a) scale down public expectations of its criminal justice arm, (b) change the criteria by which success of the state in maintaining law and order is to be judged, and (c) make crime prevention and crime control an implicit responsibility of all its citizens. Perhaps because of its legacy, psychiatry finds itself at the centre of the 'fight against crime and the causes of crime', to borrow an oft-repeated call by the British ex-prime minister, Tony Blair. It should be noted that the criminal justice state is a hypothetical notion rather than the accepted definition of any state, utilised to understand the ideological and procedural aspects of governments. This notion can be predominantly applied to policies and practices of the UK government and psychiatrists within this system, although much of this may also have relevance to other countries.

Public health psychiatry

The community 'experiment'

A public health (and safety) agenda formed the focus of psychiatry and set it aside from most other branches of medicine, even at its birth. Thus, even at the birth of modern psychiatry in France, whilst a distinction was made between immoral behaviour and mental illness,[3] the fact that the place where those exhibiting such behaviours were held was the asylum suggested a sociopolitical will to concentrate criminal behaviour in mental institutions.[4] *Manie sans delire*, was probably the earliest forerunner of antisocial personality disorder, espousing the central notion of violent and bizarre behaviour,[5] and a spate of other similar diagnoses sprang up that essentially focused upon behaviours proscribed by the society, rather than any specific pathological state that medicine could verify. Moral insanity,[6] dissolute immorality,[7] moral imbecility and constitutional psychopathic inferiority[8] all referred to a state where there was morbid perversion of behaviour. An authoritative voice of medicine at that time, Maudsley, wrote that such disorders were a 'form of mental alienation which has so much the look of vice' that 'it is an unfounded medical invention' and 'which must either be got rid of out of the social organisation or be sequestrated and made harmless in it'.[9]

Thus, the origins of psychiatry as a branch of medicine were steeped in public health concerns, and the profession historically plied its trade often in arenas removed from public view. These duties were enshrined in the earliest mental health legislations, not only in the UK, but also in its colonies.[10] The advent of modern diagnostic systems and psychotherapeutic approaches to treatment, and the development of newer pharmacological agents collectively conspired to herald the development of community treatment for the mentally ill over decades of gradual incremental changes in clinical practices. This evolution drew upon critiques of total institutions and the dangers of stigma and social exclusion,[2] and occurred largely within sociopolitical contexts of the collapse of a cult of war and feminist movements of Western Europe and North America in the mid-1970s, to name just two influential factors.[11] This represented the advent of libertarian movements and a willingness to view the mentally disordered not as the *alien other* but as one of us, and to normalise their lives. Within forensic psychiatry, the most notable case was that of Johnnie Braxtrom, a mentally ill offender. Diverted from prison into a state hospital for the criminally insane in the USA, and inadvertently detained beyond the term of his prison sentence, he successfully appealed in the Supreme Court that his constitutional rights had been violated. He, along with 966 similarly detained offender-patients, were transferred to a civil mental hospitals; the so-called Braxstrom experiment.[12] A 4-year follow-up revealed much lower than anticipated rates of offending. Of the 246 patients who had by then reached the community, only two committed serious crimes of violence.[13] This was the beginning of the community being the panacea for the mentally disordered.

However, the heady success of community experiments was dented by high-profile homicides, which, in the UK, started with the case of Christopher Clunis. Suffering with severe and treatment-resistant paranoid schizophrenia, he pushed an unknown stranger, Jonathan Zito, into the path of an oncoming train in London, in direct response to his psychotic experiences at the time. A confidential homicide inquiry, the first of a series of similar mandatory exercises that were instituted after all cases of homicide by the mentally ill, made scathing criticisms of the quality of care provided by mental health and social care providers to Mr Clunis, which heralded major changes in psychiatric practice.[14] These recommendations were enshrined in various legislations that introduced concepts such as a supervision register, mandatory risk assessments, the care programme approach, care in the community, etc – effectively establishing far-reaching control over community patients.[15] Over the next decade or so, notwithstanding occasional murmurs of discontent, psychiatrists adopted changes that included: (a) establishing links between mental disorder and offending, (b) assessing risk in a dynamic way, and (c) the development of multidisciplinary and multi-agency working. These changes imperceptibly moved psychiatric practice once again towards prioritising control over the mentally disordered, with a corresponding hardening of the public's attitude and perception of the mentally disordered.[16]

However, hospital care is expensive and the requirement to consider risks and to manage them successfully at all times had to be balanced with the need to move patients into the community within the state-run NHS (National Health Service) system. The government sought to gradually separate inpatient services from outpatient services and to ostensibly provide improved care to patients within or closer to their homes, and achieve a degree of equity in professional caseloads, which culminated in the creation of specialist teams for assertive community treatment, home treatment, early intervention, etc. For the mentally ill offender, long-term hospital treatment was not only more expensive than for the non-forensic group, it also prevented the high volume of mentally disordered prison inmates from gaining entry into scarce and expensive beds. Of individuals in prison, 10% are reported to have serious mental illness and 80% to have personality disorder.[17]

The need to empty oversubscribed forensic hospital beds at a pace commensurate with the high demand for them, meant that increasing numbers of mentally disordered offenders were being managed in the community, albeit that most were considered 'safe' at the time of their discharges. But the gains made by many of them were achieved in supportive and protected hospital environments, which could not be replicated in the community.

Whilst experience with Clunis led to increased control on those in the community, the case of Michael Stone, led to the development of the Dangerous and Severe Personality Disorder (DSPD) initiative (see below). Stone had been a personality-disordered individual who was considered untreatable under existing mental health legal definitions and was therefore discharged by psychiatrists. Within days of being discharged he had killed a mother and her daughter, leading the then home secretary Jack Straw to suggest in the House of Commons that any decent psychiatrist would have locked him up 20 years ago, whether treatable or not.[18] Not surprisingly, violent offences by the mentally disordered, stoked by adverse reports by a media[19] that had already conducted a media trial and found psychiatrists guilty of negligence,[20] made the government increasingly vulnerable to the voices of pressure groups castigating it for a perceived failure of care in the community. Although an inquiry later found that Michael Stone's care had been exemplary, politicians used such opportunities to send messages to their constituents often by 'parading' victims and their families. This was done in an attempt to divert the attention of irate constituents onto 'misguided psychiatrists' who were named and shamed,[21,22] and used to deflect attention from an overloaded system that was poorly funded and supported.

A 'criminal justice state' approach to crime management

Community remains the solution

Despite the 'accidents', the fact that the community continued to be a solution for many offenders – mentally disordered or not – is a reflection of the strategy of the criminal justice state in managing crime and prisoner numbers.[2] 'Community' in these instances merely means noncustodial and occurring outside of prisons. Similar arguments of the undesirability of total institutions, stigma and social exclusion, which had led to the community experiment within psychiatry, now facilitated moving offenders out of overcrowded prisons, whilst extolling the virtues of the healing powers of community relations. These developments found state employees rather than lay members of the community carrying out state policies, under the auspices of local authority organisation.[23] It is now common to find a community psychiatric nurse working with a patient alongside the police, probation and other local authority services in managing patients, where in actual fact the team is managing crime prevention.

The inter-agency strategy

The attempt to extend the reach of state agencies by linking them up with the practices of individual actors within the private sector (read non-criminal justice system sector) and the community (read voluntary and charitable agencies who run hostels and housing schemes) has been described as a 'responsibilization strategy'.[24] Instead of dealing with crime directly by means of police, courts, prisons and probation, this approach led to an enhanced network of formal and informal structures (e.g. visits by a social care support worker or a community mental health nurse to a forensic hostel where an ex-offender is located). This is the essence of the new crime-prevention approach that has been developed by the Anglo-American governments, the key phrases of the new strategy being terms such as 'working in partnerships', 'interagency cooperation', 'multi-agency approach', etc, which are given quasi-legal support beyond administrative directives, through recommendations within homicide inquiries into the care of mental health patients.[22] In this manner, the individual professional is coerced by the various arms of the governments and the society it represents. Mental health legislation incorporated and created new categories and processes to enforce treatment in the community, section 25(a) supervision orders,[15] multiagency public-protection arrangements, and treatments for sex offenders, provided within a network of professionals.

Redistributing the task of crime control, rendering others responsible, multiplying the number of effective authorities, forming alliances, arranging things so that crime-control duties follow crime-generating behaviours – these are the new and institutionally radical goals that are now being pursued. The criminal justice state is, in this area at least, shedding its 'sovereign' style of governing by top-down command and developing a form of rule close to that described by Michel Foucault as governmentality – a modality that involves the enlistment of others, the shaping of incentives, and the creation of new forms of cooperative actions.[25]

Redefining success

Police in many countries now generally hold low expectations for the control of crimes, the great majority of which they now refer to as random and opportunistic offending.[2] Similarly, prisons focus on their ability to hold offenders securely in custody thus incapacitating and/or punishing them. They are circumspect in claiming the capacity to produce rehabilitative effects, transferring the rehabilitative functions to newly developed pilots of management of such offenders,[2] or not providing rehabilitation at all.[26] One such pilot is the UK governments Dangerous and Severe Personality Disorder (DSPD) programme.[27] This collective venture brings together the Ministry of Justice, the Department of Health, the Prison Service and the NHS, to deliver new mental health services for people who are, or have previously been, considered dangerous, due to a functional link between dangerousness and severe personality disorder. The programme currently runs pilot projects **(expected to be concluded in 2014)** in four units opened at Broadmoor and Rampton maximum secure hospitals, and Frankland and Whitemoor maximum secure prisons, assessing and treating offenders who meet the DSPD criteria. Similar programmes already exist in the USA under their Sexual Predator and Dangerous Offender laws, and the Dangerous Prisoners (Sexual Offenders) Act 2003, in the state of Queensland in Australia.

The DSPD programme's importance can be gauged by the fact that it was included in the last labour Government's manifesto and is described by the official DSPD website as

> a ground breaking initiative aimed at supporting public protection through the development of pilot treatment services for dangerous offenders whose offending is linked to severe personality disorder. It is aimed at people who have committed a violent and/or sexual crime and have been detained under the criminal justice system or current mental health legislation.

By an unknown process, the government calculated that there were about 400 males (the programme does not extend to women yet) who 'suffered' from this condition, and referred to them as 'some of the most difficult and dangerous persons in society'. While there are explicit criteria denoting those who are appropriate for admission to the DSPD services, there are no corresponding criteria to identify those who should leave. It has been suggested that there are few empirical data to inform clinical decision making on the level of risk, and the impact of interventions thought to reduce risk that such individuals might pose on release from high secure services.[28]

Additionally, most treatment programmes for personality-disordered offenders in the UK, whether carried out within prisons or in the mental health system, are not underpinned by an adequately powered evidence base.[29] It is likely that individuals designated as DSPD will make slow progress to lower levels of security unless these gaps in knowledge are addressed.[28] Nevertheless, it is only a matter of time until such pilot programmes become the rehabilitative and 'long-term management arm' of the prison services,[2] despite shortcomings in the entire process.

Reinventing mental health and criminal justice legislation

Whilst efficacy data of experimental strategies to reduce future risks of harm to the public is the desired Holy Grail, notwithstanding the extent to which these would translate into effectiveness data, the criminal justice states have already created categories of offenders who it is hoped benefit from interventions. It has also created new performance indicators that are designed to measure 'outputs' rather than 'outcomes'. These indicators measure what an individual or organisation does rather than what, if anything, it achieves. Hence, the shift of sentencing policy towards mandatory penalties, sentencing guidelines, and just desserts has the effect of focusing attention firmly upon process and away from outcome. For judges, it shifts sentencing away from a focus on reduction in crime through individualised sentencing to fitting the punishment to the offence, i.e. fixed sentences where there is no scope for being innovative or creative. Until 2003, psychiatrists in the UK were asked to provide dangerousness assessments under section 2(2b) of the Criminal Justice Act 1991.[30] The level of future risk or dangerousness was derived from psychiatric (or other professionals', e.g. probation officers') testimony and *not* automatically assumed by the sentencing judges. Psychiatrists could choose to remain outside this process, invoking ethical and other reasons.[31]

This changed when the Criminal Justice Act 2003 created a new category of offender – the dangerous offender – where for those who are older than 18 years of age and have previous convictions, there is a *statutory assumption of significant risk in future to members of public*. These provisions termed DOP or dangerous offender provisions led to the Indeterminate Public Protection order or IPP, which leads to an automatic life sentence under section 225 of the Criminal Justice Act 2003. However, mental health act orders under section 37 (MHA 1983) will override the dangerous offender provisions and, as such, there is an *automatic requirement of psychiatric assessment* of the offender's mental condition and a functional link between this and a future risk of significant harm to members of public. In *R. v. Lang and others*,[32] the court established criteria against which future significant risk should be assessed, and advised that the following factors should routinely be taken into account: (a) the nature and circumstances of the current offence, (b) a past history of offending, the relevant circumstances and sentences passed, (c) whether offending demonstrated a pattern, (d) social and economic factors such as accommodation, employability, education, associates, relationships, drug and alcohol abuse, (e) current and past emotional state, and (f) the offender's attitude towards offending and supervision. Since the government made DOP and IPP mandatory, giving judges no discretion over sentencing, contrary to government estimates of around 900 convictions, there are now close to 3000 convictions, with many prisoners languishing in prisons even after their tariff (the duration of imprisonment which their last offence would have attracted) has expired. This has led to legal challenges.[26] It is anticipated that some of these individuals will be transferred to mental health facilities that specialise in providing treatment to those with antisocial personality disorder,[29,33] and some units now specialise in doing so.[28]

It is perhaps no accident that these changes to sentencing laws have neatly dovetailed with the DSPD pilots which started around the same time. The Department of Health's documents suggest that psychiatrists can no longer use diagnoses of personality disorder to exclude patients from treatment.[34] It is thought that the criminal justice government does such things as a first step in identifying people or organisations thought to have competence and expertise in assessing and effectively reducing criminal propensities and opportunities. It also assesses which agencies have a direct responsibility to do so (criminal justice agencies) and whether this responsibility can be enforced.[35] Whatever the underlying reasons for the assumption that psychiatrists are experts in crime management and prevention, the strategies discussed mean that psychiatrists and mental health services are a key part of government measures to ensure public safety.

It is also no coincidence that the revisions to the Mental Health Act (2007) for England and Wales, removed the treatability clause of the Mental Health Act 1983, the one crucial factor that had hitherto allowed psychiatrists the legal justification of not treating unmotivated personality-disordered individuals, especially those who harm others, in involuntary detention. The most controversial aspects of this legislation include firstly a broader definition of mental disorder. This can be any disorder or disability of mind, removing the existing four categories and including promiscuity, immoral conduct and sexual deviancy, such that not only is a larger group of individuals detained, but even those who are sexually deviant without even being personality disordered can now be detained involuntarily. Secondly, the treatability clause is removed. It is no longer necessary to demonstrate that there is any therapeutic benefit to medical treatment, which can be given under compulsion merely to treat the symptoms or manifestations of the disorder without the disorder itself being judged to be curable or treatable. Finally, community treatment orders that will set conditions to enforce individuals to accept treatments, failing which they would be liable to be returned to hospital without the need for 're-sectioning', effectively extends the reach of mental health law into the homes of patients, and perhaps forever alters the quality and dynamic of the patient–professional relationship.[36]

New performance markers

Criminal justice states have simultaneously created new performance indicators for assessing the effectiveness of mental healthcare services.

Performances of organisations are increasingly measured in terms of the number of patients assessed, admitted or discharged, the frequency and intensity of input of various members of care teams,[37] the number of hours that patients in hospitals (and inmates in prison) spend in purposeful or meaningful activity, and so on.[38] Performances are not measured in terms of whether they bring about resolution of objectively assessed needs or reduce subsequent offending.[39] Similarly, nursing staff are judged according to the number of nurses on shift (similar to police officers on beat), the number of critical incidents generated and complaints processed, the speed of response following an incident/complaint, or some other measure of economy and efficiency of the organisation rather than any tangible benefit on patient outcomes or reduction in rates of criminal convictions.[33,40] In tandem, discourses of these agencies seek to shift responsibility for outcomes onto their customers, thereby offsetting organisational liability. The mental health patient, unless he is floridly psychotic, is now said to be responsible for making use of any rehabilitative opportunities in hospital or in the community, and is usually expected to sign a contract accepting responsibility for adhering to a prescribed code of conduct and recommended treatment, as requirements within the care programme approach. There is a similar expectation from offenders on probation or community service.

Concentration on consequences

There is a recent trend of concentrating on consequences rather than causes of crime, and remediation by criminal justice agencies. Thus the harmful effects of criminal conduct are routinely addressed by supporting victims, and addressing public fear and insecurity,[41] the latter through diversion of public attention onto their own members, i.e. hapless psychiatrists who are publicly denigrated,[21,22] and deflecting attention from an overloaded system that is poorly funded and supported. In order to instil a sense of empowerment, victims are now expected to be closely involved in a patient's ongoing treatment and detention, and have a say in the discharge planning through representation at mental health review tribunals as envisaged in the Domestic Violence, Crime and Victims Act 2004.[42] To reflect these concerns, multi-agency public-protection arrangements meetings now regularly incorporate victims' issues to determine whether patients can be relocated and access services in their home areas to which they may have belonged, or where family and other supports are available.

Is assessing and treating future violence a psychiatric 'duty'?

How are psychiatrists to deal with the ethical ramifications of being directly involved in state-sponsored crime-reduction and management programmes? As members of a democratic society where the people and their elected representatives clearly hold psychiatrists responsible for risk removal, what evidence can they resort to in establishing firstly whether they really possess particular skills that no one else has; secondly the limits to which their expertise is owned by the state for its own use; and thirdly, whether the ethical principles that govern them as members of the medical profession allow them to effectively do harm to their patients by perpetuating their detention without a clear benefit to the patient.

Is dangerousness a psychiatric construct?

The causes of criminal activity are so diverse and widespread, being features of social pathologies within a society and the society's level of tolerance of perceived deviance from societal norms, that to separately relate offences to abnormal mental capacities and functions is probably disingenuous. It has been shown that the risk factors for crime amongst both the individuals who are mentally disordered and those who are not, are the same.[13] However, by invoking the label of personality disorder, society can absolve itself of its direct responsibility in creating some of these social pathologies and lay the blame firmly at the feet of the 'offender', now labelled as the 'patient', and giving the responsibility for controlling his deviant behaviours to professionals.

Defining a mental disorder in terms of perceived dangerousness, rather than the psychological and functional impairment of the individual, was previously enshrined in the Fallon Report,[43] which defined severe personality disorder as 'individuals who both suffer from a personality disorder or disorders, one of which will generally be antisocial personality disorder, and who pose a risk of causing serious harm to others'. This raises the moot question; is 'dangerousness' a medical diagnosis, and in conducting risk assessments are psychiatrists conducting legitimate medical investigations? Dangerousness has been defined as 'a propensity to cause serious physical illness or lasting psychological harm' by the Butler Committee,[44] and as 'an unpredictable and untreatable tendency to inflict or risk irreversible injury or destruction or to induce others to do so'. Both definitions view dangerousness as a static or permanent feature of a person's psyche. In reality, violence is a dynamic relationship; interplay between proximate persons and circumstances, best demonstrated by the equation: 'offender + victim + circumstances = offence'.[45] A person may be violent with a victim possessing a particular profile in a particular context, and yet may be entirely appropriately behaved at other times and with those who do not fit this profile.

Psychiatrists are already involved in predicting future violence, yet an extensive but dated review reveals that for every three patients detained by psychiatrists on the grounds of future risk, only one would subsequently commit a violent act, and that the best predictor of future violence is the same for offenders who are mentally disordered or not, i.e. a history of previous violence.[46,47] A more recent study reports that six people would have to be detained preventatively (or prophylactically) to prevent one violent act, and that making short-term risk predictions does not improve the accuracy.[48] A concept of dangerousness therefore appears to be a criminological and not a medical concept, but, more importantly, psychiatrists are not experts in the reliable assessment of the future risk of violence.

Mental health professionals now make use of various psychometric risk instruments, which many feel allow more reliable opinions to be expressed about the risk of violence. However, such instruments are actuarial in nature, i.e. they predict risk of future violence by particular *groups* of people. Although such methods allow more reliable predictions, they ignore individual variations in risk, focus on relatively static variables, fail to prioritise clinically relevant variables, and minimise the role of professional judgement. As a result of its promise to differentiate between those likely to be violent in the future from those who will not be so, the revised version of the Psychopathy Checklist (PCL-R) is widely regarded as one of the best instruments available,[49] and is widely used in the criminal justice system in the UK, the USA and Europe. It is claimed, worryingly, that the PCL-R explains only 7% of the behaviours that it seeks to predict, and fails to differentiate adequately between violent and non-violent offenders.[50] Freedman also warns that, given the high false-positive rates, the PCL-R should not be used in forensic settings or clinical settings where life and liberty decisions are made.[50] Even then, new best practice guidance regarding risk-assessment tools for assessing risk of violence, sexual violence, and antisocial and offending behaviour in the UK, identify the PCL-R, along with the Historical Clinical Risk-20 (HCR-20),[51] and the Violence Risk Appraisal Guide (VRAG),[52] as some of the most reliable tools available.[53] Some of these instruments contain items that assess risk in a dynamic way, reflecting a desirable shift in government policies away from static actuarial risk ratings (i.e. a categorical view of dangerousness) to structured clinical judgements where both static and dynamic risk factors are utilised in risk predictions.[54]

Who 'owns' psychiatric expertise?

Psychiatrists have a lot to offer in assessing dynamic aspects of risk, especially with those who have serious mental illnesses. Thus, psychotic symptoms, agitated depression, manic aggression, substance and alcohol abuse, for example, are aspects of dynamic risk that the psychiatrist is trained to advise on. However, psychiatrists can struggle with assessing risk in those with personality disorders, for it is a stable and relatively inflexible aspect of one's personhood and has not been demonstrated to co-vary with offending.[29] Correlation between offending and antisocial personality disorder[17] suffers from the problem of tautology – the behaviour is the disorder and the disorder is the behaviour. Should psychiatrists therefore restrict themselves to advising merely on those aspects of dynamic risk assessment that they have expertise in conducting? This would have the advantage of identifying only those psychiatric and psychosocial factors that can be manipulated through interventions, and would therefore ensure that a welfare purpose is served. This is most relevant whilst advising courts of future risk.

More importantly, advising on risk issues does not make a psychiatrist the most skilled professional to treat the risk of violence, especially when this is carried out under compulsory powers. Indeed, most treatments used within an institutional setting in the NHS to reduce recidivism have been created within penal institutions in North America by forensic psychologists, criminologists and those working within the criminal justice system.[29] If such provisions are accepted voluntarily by patients then there is no ethical dilemma. The problem arises when psychiatrists become responsible for causing longer than commensurate sentences,[31] or indeterminate life sentences for prisoners,[55] and then detaining them as patients under mental health legislation.

But does the state have a valid claim on medical expert testimony? It is difficult to argue that it does not. The state takes an active interest in the regulation of doctors, particularly in the UK where nearly all aspects of forensic and most parts of general mental health care are conducted under policies and targets established by the state. However, as past experience of Nazi doctors and those in the Soviet Union has shown, there is widespread condemnation of medical expertise being used for political purposes. In fact the government's proposals have been seen as proposals for preventive detention, intended to circumvent the European Convention on Human Rights, which prohibits preventive detention except in those of unsound mind.[56] Given the above, it is imperative that ethically grounded practice should routinely involve an explanation by the psychiatrist to the person assessed, of the parameters of their meeting. The appraisee may find it difficult to treat the doctor as anything other than a doctor, and these considerations argue powerfully for a separation between the evaluation and treatment roles. Within the British system of catchment area psychiatry, this is probably impossible to achieve.[57]

Ethical considerations

Psychiatrists are first and foremost doctors and should work within the ethical standards that govern the medical profession, most notably the principles of 'beneficence' and 'non-maleficence', i.e. *doing good* and *avoiding harm*.[58] The UK Royal College of Psychiatrists has provided guidance for psychiatrists and members of the college on adopting various ethical positions in order to ethically justify and rationalise their actions.[57] One argument is that by detaining and treating the patient, the psychiatrist is helping the patient, which otherwise would not have been possible. Secondly, when treatment is not available, as a citizen of a state that conforms to the European Convention of Human Rights which states that there is a human right to be protected from a known risk from others, within a public health perspective the psychiatrist has a duty to advise courts about future risks and their functional link to mental disorder/s, even if no treatment can be provided. Under the revisions of the Mental Health Act (2007) for England and Wales, the psychiatrist is responsible for detaining high-risk individuals and treating them in the hope that this would be effective, even if no evidence-based effective treatment may exist currently. This may force the question should I be involved in such a system? The Royal College report suggests that there are potentially four ways in which this question can be answered, and ethical justifications are provided for each of the positions adopted.

The psychiatrist can adopt the traditional medical ethics model of beneficence and non-maleficence as one extreme stance and refuse to be involved in even assessing individuals, unless there is a welfare disposal, i.e. there is some scintilla of benefit to the individual. A further extension of this position is to only act for the defence when the assessment is clearly within a framework of potential benefit to the patient. At the other extreme, the psychiatrist can become involved as a pure 'forensicist', i.e. in doing so they are not acting as a doctor but as a risk specialist who can give evidence that could lead to enhanced punishment.[59] In between these poles, the psychiatrist can choose to operate from the framework of justice ethics, i.e. it is in everybody's interests that there is good quality evidence available to the court in relation to making just decisions.

Protection for patients

It has been argued that when legal and medical values clash, particularly in the domain of mental health, medical values and objectives should take precedence over legal ones, not least because the legal process can cause 'juridogenic harm' to patients.[60] However, there are different constructions of the word 'good'. Legal ethics emphasise respect for autonomy and liberty, whilst medical ethics tend to privilege beneficence and healthy paternalism, where a 'good' outcome means 'what is good clinically'. Doctors tend to operate on the beneficence principle that has traditionally been paternalistic, but as there was a best *medical* interest principle, society allowed a fair degree of paternalism. But the House of Lords in *F. v. West Berkshire Health Authority* held that liberty and respect for autonomy may mean more to the patient than their medical health,[61] a point since made repeatedly in courts that have assessed individuals' competence to refuse treatment. Should consideration be given to risk assessments being a medical investigation if psychiatrists are to be made responsible for it, and should it require the same rigour in obtaining full consent, as the procedure could conceivably carry significant risks of harm to the patient in terms of loss of liberty and autonomy?[56]

But in psychiatry, 'best interests' is often conflated with 'best *social* interests', in terms of duties to third parties in the prevention of harm, and mental health legislation in many countries incorporates risk of harm to others as one of the major reasons for compulsory detention. Psychiatrists testifying at mental health tribunals currently have a dual function in that they act as agents for the health authority and, by extension, the patient, and also as agents with a responsibility for public safety. If the dual agency were made explicit from the start, this particular harm of one's doctor's actions, often in the bests interest of third parties, could be minimised. Better still, this harm to the therapeutic alliance could be avoided altogether by separating the therapeutic and legal roles of the psychiatrist. There would be the benefit of increased transparency about the roles of the psychiatrist and the avoidance of bias. The knowledge that one's treating psychiatrist has this duty from some unclear public mandate might cause patients to believe that s/he does not have their interests as a first concern, and to turn to their lawyers. This may not be 'juridogenic harm'; if anything it is an 'iatrogenic harm'. This mistrust of doctors may explain why many patients are increasingly using tribunals as a type of case review, where the clinical judgment of the consultant psychiatrist is questioned, although that is not the intended purpose of tribunals. Similarly, doctors sometimes use a tribunal's recommendation to press the Ministry of Justice for a particular desired outcome, usually in collusion with the patient's lawyers.

Loyalty is a key value for the lawyer in the pursuit of justice for his client and this may necessitate withholding unfavourable reports, an action consistent with Article 5 of the Human Rights Act 1998 that guarantees a right to protection against self-incrimination. Most people seek to protect their own interests above those of others of society, and the mentally disordered should not be expected to be more altruistic. As such, tribunals act to regulate the tension between the individual and societal interests. There is no right to treatment derived either from common law or the Human Rights Act (1998), but a right to liberty exists in both. Consequently, expecting tribunals to base their rulings on solely therapeutic considerations in preference to natural laws of justice is unrealistic, and represents the tension that psychiatrists experience and must balance in terms of whether or not they are agents of the state or agents for their patients. At the present time, this boundary is blurred.[62]

Conclusions

Psychiatrists are both doctors and citizens of their states and are therefore subject to ethical standards and moral duties that can conflict with each other. Their patients are often prisoners in disguise and traverse the thin line between paternalistic beneficence and preventative detention. They look to the psychiatrist when they have committed serious offences, to divert them into the mental health system, and when there, seek assistance of lawyers to gain a rapid re-entry into the society through the 'back door'. The competing and conflicting clinical, legal and ethical tensions that psychiatrists and their patients experience within a framework of 'care' and 'control', are dialectics that will reverberate for many years to come.

Key learning points

1. Forensic psychiatry is increasingly required to ensure public safety following high profile 'failures of the community care' of patients who pose risk of harm to others

2. The UK government, by adopting a 'culture of control' has amended mental health & criminal justice legislations, places psychiatrists at the centre of its crime prevention and control measures.
3. All psychiatrists must take an appropriate and satisfactory ethical position when asked to act on the state's behalf in order to minimise iatrogenic and juridogenic harm to the doctor-patient relationship.

References

1. Shorter E. *A History of Psychiatry.* New York: John Wiley, 1997, p. 341.
2. Garland D. *The Culture of Control – Crime and Social Order in Contemporary Society.* Oxford: Oxford University Press; 2002.
3. Lopez-Ibor J. Introduction to personality disorders. In: Gelder MG, Lopez-Ibor JJ, Andreasen NC, editors. *New Oxford Textbook of Psychiatry.* Oxford: Oxford University Press; 2000, p. 919.
4. Morel BA. *Traite des Degenerescences Physiques, Intellectuelles et Morales de l'Espece Humaine.* JB Baillière ; 1839.
5. Pinel P. *Traite Medico-philosophique sur L'Alienaiton Mentale.* Richard Caille et Ravier; 1801.
6. Prichard JC. *A Treatise on Insanity.* London: Sherwood, Gilbert, and Piper; 1835.
7. Lewis A. Psychopathic personality: a most elusive category. *Psychological Medicine* 1974 4: 133–40.
8. Henderson D, Gillespie RD. *A Textbook of Psychiatry,* 3rd edn. London: Oxford University Press; 1932
9. Maudsley H. *Responsibility in Mental Disease.* London: Kind; 1874
10. Sarkar J, Dutt AB. Forensic psychiatry in India: time to wake up. *Journal of Forensic Psychiatry and Psychology* 2006; 17: 121–30.
11. Herman J. *Trauma and Recovery.* New York: Basic Books; 1992.
12. Steadman HJ, Cocozza J. *Careers of the Criminally Insane.* Lexington: Lexington Books; 1974.
13. Chiswick D. Dangerousness. In: Chiswick D, Cope R, editors. *Practical Forensic Psychiatry.* London: Gaskell, Royal College of Psychiatrists; 1995, pp. 210–242.
14. Ritchie J, Dick D, Lingham R. *The Report of the Inquiry into the Care and Treatment of Christopher Clunis.* London: TSO (The Stationery Office); 1994.
15. Eastman N. The Mental Health (Patients in the Community) Act 1995: a clinical analysis. *British Journal of Psychiatry* 1997; 170: 492–6.
16. Ministers act on mental care. Homeless former hospital patient an affront to society, Heseltine says. *The Independent* 20 January 1992.
17. Singleton N, Meltzer H, Gatward R, Coid J, Deasy D. *Psychiatry Morbidity among Prisoners in England and Wales.* London: The Stationery Office; 1998.
18. Wessley S. You can't just lock up psychopaths. *The Independent* 29 October 1998.
19. Court C. Clunis inquiry cites 'catalogue of failures'. *BMJ* 1994; 308: 613.
20. Gaber I. How the big Michael Stone story was missed. *The Guardian* 2 October 2006. www.guardian.co.uk/media/2006/oct/02/mondaymedia section.socialcare (accessed 22 March 2011).

21. Cavendish C. They are getting away with murder: mental health services are in turmoil. *The Times* 23 November 2006. www.timesonline.co.uk/tol/comment/columnists/camilla_cavendish/article646406.ece (accessed 22 March 2011).
22. South West London Strategic Health Authority. *Independent Inquiry into the Care and Treatment of John Barrett.* London: NHS Publications; 2006.
23. Karp DR. *Community Justice: an emerging field.* Lanham: Rowman and Littlefield; 1998.
24. O'Malley P. Risk, power and crime prevention. *Economy and Society* 1992, 21: 252–75.
25. Foucault M. *'Govermentality' in The Foucault Effect.* New York: Harvester Wheatsheaf; 1992.
26. Dyer C. Ministers face legal challenge over jails crisis. *The Guardian* 4 June 2007. www.guardian.co.uk/uk_news/story/0,,2094683,00.html (accessed 22 March 2011).
27. Home Office and Department of Health. *Managing Dangerous People with Severe Personality Disorder. Proposals for policy development.* London: Home Office and Department of Health; 1999.
28. Duggan C. To move or not to move – that is the question! Some reflections on the transfer of DSPD patients in the face of uncertainty. *Psychology Crime and Law* 2007; 13: 113–21.
29. Howells K, Krishnan G, Daffern M. Challenges in the treatment of dangerous and severe personality disorders. *Advances in Psychiatric Treatment* 2007; 13: 325–32.
30. Thomas D. *Sentencing News* 1994; 4: 8–11
31. Solomka B. The role of psychiatric evidence in passing 'longer than normal' sentences. *Journal of Forensic Psychiatry* 1996; 7: 239–55.
32. *R. v. Lang* [2005]. http://www.bailii.org/ew/cases/EWCA/Crim/2005/2864.html
33. Davies S, Clarke M, Hollin C, Duggan C. Long-term outcomes after discharge from medium secure care: a cause for concern. *British Journal of Psychiatry* 2007; 191: 70–4.
34. Department of Health. *Personality Disorder: no longer a diagnosis of exclusion.* London: Department of Health; 2003.
35. Hough M. Introduction. In: Clarke R, Mayhew P, editors. *Designing out Crime.* London: HMSO; 1980.
36. Department of Health. *Mental Health Act 1983* [to be amended by the Mental Health Act 2007]. London: Department of Health; 2007.
37. Department of Health. *New Ways of Working for Everyone: a best practice implementation guide.* London: Department of Health; 2007.
38. Her Majesty's Prison Service. *Framework Document.* London: Prison Service; 1999.
39. King RD, McDermott K. *The State of our Prisons.* Oxford: Oxford University Press; 1995.
40. Maden A, Scott F, Burdett R. Offending in psychiatric patients after discharge from medium secure units: prospective national cohort study. *BMJ* 2004; 328: 1534.
41. Home Office. *A Review of Criminal Justice Policy.* London: HMSO; 1976.
42. Domestic Violence Crime and Victims Act 2004. www.opsi.gov.uk/ACTS/acts2004/ukpga_20040028_en_1 (accessed 22 March 2011).

43. Department of Health. *Report of the Committee of Inquiry into the Personality Disorder Unit, Ashworth Special Hospital.* Cm 4194-11. London: The Stationery Office; 1999.
44. Home Office and Department of Health and Social Security. *Report of the Committee in Mentally Abnormal Offenders (Butler Report).* Cmnd 6244. London: HMSO; 1975.
45. Scott PD. Assessing dangerousness in criminals. *British Journal of Psychiatry* 1977; 131: 127–42.
46. Monahan J. The prediction of violent behaviour: toward a second generation of theory and policy. *American Journal of Psychiatry* 1984; 141: 10–15.
47. Monahan J. Dangerousness: an American perspective. In: Gunn J, Taylor PJ, editors. *Forensic Psychiatry: clinical, legal and ethical issues.* Oxford: Butterworth Heinemann; 1993, pp. 624–645.
48. Buchanan A, Leese M. Detention of people with dangerous severe personality disorders: a systematic review. *Lancet* 2001; 358: 1955–8.
49. Hare RD. *The Hare Psychopathy Checklist – Revised.* Toronto: Multi-Health Systems; 1991.
50. Freedman D. False prediction of future dangerousness: error rates and Psychopathy Checklist-Revised. *Journal of the American Academy of Psychiatry and the Law* 2001, 29: 89–95.
51. Webster CD, Douglas KS, Eaves D, Hart D. *HCR-20. Assessing Risk for Violence, Version 2.* Vancouver: Mental Health, Law and Policy Institute, Simon Fraser University; 1997.
52. Quinsey V, Harris G, Rice M, Cormier C. *Violent Offenders: appraising and managing risk.* Washington DC: American Psychological Association. 1998.
53. Coid J, Yang M, Ulrich S et al. *Predicting and Understanding Risk of Re-offending: The Prisoner Cohort Study.* London: Ministry of Justice; 2007.
54. Maden T. *Treating Violence.* Oxford: Oxford University Press; 2007.
55. Criminal Justice Act 2003. www.opsi.gov.uk/acts/acts2003/ukpga_20030044_en_1 (accessed 22 March 2011).
56. Eastman N. Public health psychiatry or crime prevention? *BMJ* 1999; 318: 549–51.
57. Royal College of Psychiatrists. *Good Psychiatric Practice,* 2nd edn. (council reports CR125). London: Royal College of Psychiatrists, 2004.
58. Weinstock R & Gold L. (2004). 'Ethics in Forensic Psychiatry' in Eds R Simon & Gold L, *Forensic Psychiatry: The Clinician's Guide.* American Psychiatric Publishing, Washington DC, pp. 91–115.
59. Stone AA. The ethical boundaries of forensic psychiatry – a view from the ivory tower. *Bulletin of the American Academy of Psychiatry and the Law* 1984; 12: 209–19.
60. Obomanu W, Kennedy H. 'Juridogenic' harm: statutory principles for the new mental health tribunals. *Psychiatric Bulletin* 2001; 25: 331–3.
61. *F. v. West Berkshire Health Authority* [1990] 2 A.C.1, http://lawiki.org/lawwiki/F_v_West_Berkshire_Health_Authority.
62. Sarkar SP, Adshead G. Black robes and white coats: who will win the new mental health tribunals? *British Journal of Psychiatry* 2005; 186

3
Younger People with Dementia

Kate Jefferies, Robert Lawrence and Niruj Agrawal

Clinical convention describes dementia as young onset if the illness starts before the age of 65 years. This precise threshold is largely arbitrary, but it attempts to highlight the pathologies of cortical neurodegeneration with differing clinical profiles, intensity of symptoms, and expected duration of disease depending on age at onset. Rarer and familial forms of dementia, in fact, tend to manifest in younger rather than in older adults.

Dementia in younger people carries a high burden of age-related and stage-of-life-specific psychosocial implications. Diagnosis, and the symptoms of the conditions, impact on individuals in middle age, often still at work and with younger families. Spouses of patients with young-onset dementia are stressed by multiple concerns, including worries about finances, their own health, and the feeling and experience of lack of support and social isolation.[1]

It is important that both younger and older patients with dementia, and their carers, receive prompt assessment, information and follow-up. Focal and systemic treatable causes of dementia and primary cortical neurodegenerations must be identified. Consideration of appropriate and careful genetic counselling applies to familial forms.

Differences between those with young-onset dementias and dementias of later life

Younger people often have different needs and commitments than older people. Younger people are more likely to be in work at the time of diagnosis, have dependent family or children, be physically fit and active, and have heavy financial commitments such as a mortgage. They are also more likely to have a rarer or familial form of dementia. Therefore, they need bespoke services to meet their specific needs. This includes: explanation of the diagnosis, provision of relevant information about sources of help and support, introduction to peer support groups and provision of information about the likely prognosis and options for packages of care. Appropriate referrals should be made to help with fears and worries, distress, and practical and financial issues that may affect the person and their carers. The person's individual, personal and social needs should be paramount in the planning of care provision.

However, provision of specialist young-onset dementia services is patchy and patients often fall between stools. Carers and sufferers often find themselves being passed from 'pillar to post' between psychiatry and neurology and also between adult, old age and liaison psychiatry services.[2] The responsibility for identifying and accessing the help that is available is often left with the carers.

Prevalence of young-onset dementias

Although dementia is predominantly a disorder of later life, there are 18,500 cases of young-onset dementia in the UK. Between the ages of 30 and 64 years, there are 78.2 cases per 100,000 males and 56.4 cases per 100,000 females. The number of people with young-onset dementia increases sharply with age (Figure 3.1). Two-thirds of all cases occur in people aged 55 years and over. Dementia affects all social and ethnic groups.

Distribution of diagnosis in young-onset dementia compared with dementia occurring later in life

The distribution of diagnoses of dementia differs between older and younger patient groups. (Figures 3.2 and 3.3). Alzheimer's disease is the commonest cause of dementia in both, but is twice as common in older people compared to younger people. Frontotemporal dementia occurs much more commonly in younger compared to older populations. Also, other rarer causes of dementia occur with greater frequency in the younger population.

Clinical approach to assessment

Assessment should be multidisciplinary. It is a process rather than a single event, the aims being to reach a diagnosis and to communicate that diagnosis to the patient and their carers. Early diagnosis is essential

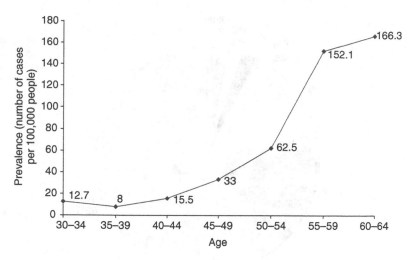

Figure 3.1 Prevalence of dementia by age

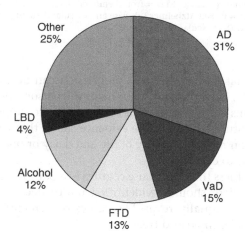

Figure 3.2 Distribution of diagnoses in young-onset dementia[3]

Notes: AD = Alzheimer's disease; Alcohol = alcohol-related dementias; FTD = frontotemporal dementia; LBD = dementia with Lewy bodies; VaD = vascular dementias.

Diagnoses that fall into the 'other' category include Huntington's disease, multiple sclerosis, Creutzfeldt–Jakob disease, Parkinson's disease, corticobasal degeneration, Down's syndrome and carbon monoxide poisoning.

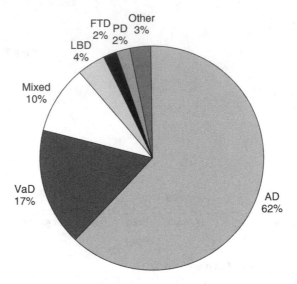

Figure 3.3   Distribution of diagnosis of dementia occurring in later life[4]

Notes: AD = Alzheimer's disease; FTD = frontotemporal dementia; LBD = dementia with Lewy bodies; Mixed = mixed Alzheimer's disease and vascular dementia; PD = Parkinson's disease dementia; VaD = vascular dementia.

so treatment that may slow illness progression can be commenced as soon as possible. Early diagnosis also helps the person and their family to come to terms with the illness, access appropriate support and make plans for the future. The available evidence shows that early diagnosis and intervention improve quality of life and delay or prevent unnecessary admissions to care homes.[5]

Psychiatric illness that may cause cognitive impairments, for example depressive disorders, should be identified and treated. Other treatable, and therefore potentially reversible, causes of dementia or delirium should also be identified and treated.

History

A history should be obtained from the patient and collateral information should be obtained from an informant. An informant's account can often provide vital information that holds the key to an accurate diagnosis.

Particular areas to be concentrated on during the history taking are: onset and evolution of symptoms, pattern of deficits, fluctuations in mental state, other past or present neurological symptoms, other current psychiatric symptoms, previous psychiatric history, past medical history, family medical and psychiatric history, use of drugs and alcohol and risk assessment.

Cognitive testing

Detailed neuropsychological testing is a helpful component of the diagnostic process. Neuropsychological testing can also help in teasing out if there has been any progression of dementia. By using a series of tests, the neuropsychologist establishes the cognitive abilities of the person and compares them to the person's estimated best levels and to those for an average person of the same age. These tests also identify where a person's abilities are preserved, so these areas can be supported and maximised.

Basic bedside testing is also helpful in confirming the nature, degree and location of deficits. The mini mental state examination (MMSE) is the most widely used screening test for cognitive impairment.[6] It is short, easy to use, has high inter-rater reliability and is useful for monitoring the progression of illness. However, it is insensitive to frontal lobe disorders, does not detect focal cognitive deficits and is strongly influenced by previous IQ and education.

The Addenbrooke's Cognitive Examination (ACE) is a more comprehensive screening instrument that contains tests of frontal lobe functioning.[7] It contains a 100-point test battery that assesses six cognitive domains. It takes about 15–20 minutes to complete and encompasses the MMSE.

For further examples of bedside tests of frontal lobe function see Table 3.1.

Table 3.1 Bedside tests of frontal lobe function

Bedside tests of frontal lobe function	Example
Verbal fluency	'Name as many words as you can beginning with the letter "S", any words except names of people or places'
Similarities	'In what way are a table and a chair alike?' 'In what way are a banana and an apple alike?'
Cognitive estimates	'How many camels are there in Holland?' 'How far is it from London to Paris?'
Proverb interpretation	'What do you understand by the saying "a rolling stone gathers no moss"?'
Luria sequence	Perform the Luria sequence 'fist-edge-palm' and ask the patient to copy it
Go-no-go test	'Tap once when I tap once. Do not tap when I tap twice'

Physical examination

Physical examination is also an essential component of the assessment of younger and older people with dementia, both in reaching the specific diagnosis of the subtype of dementia and in identifying any treatable comorbidity.

The physical examination is often unremarkable in the early stages of dementia, but the presence of certain symptoms and signs should arouse suspicion of a primary neurological disorder. These include sudden onset of symptoms, focal neurological findings early in the illness, visual hallucinations, incontinence, ataxia and early seizures.

In Alzheimer's disease, patients are typically physically well with no neurological signs in the early stages. Later there may be akinesia and rigidity. In frontotemporal dementia, neurological signs are also typically absent in the early stages. Later there may be evidence of primitive reflexes (Table 3.2) and with further disease progression there may be akinesia and rigidity. Spontaneous features of parkinsonism are one of the core features of dementia with Lewy bodies. Huntington's disease is evidenced by the presence of chorea and other pyramidal signs. In Creutzfeldt–Jakob disease (CJD), myoclonus and other extrapyramidal signs are often present.

It is worth noting that these are not diagnostic of frontal lobe damage, as they can occur in the normal elderly population, but their presence is suggestive of frontal lobe disease.

Investigations

When arranging for further investigations, the priorities are to identify treatable causes of dementia and to guide accurate diagnosis.

Table 3.2   Primitive reflexes

Reflex	Explanation
Grasp reflex	Involuntary gripping of objects in patient's hands or feet
Snout reflex	Puckering of the lips in response to tapping of the upper or lower lip
Palmomental reflex	Ipsilateral contraction of the mentalis muscle in response to stroking of the thenar eminence of the hand

The authors would suggest that the following investigations are carried out routinely

- full blood count
- erythrocyte sedimentation rate
- C-reactive protein
- renal function
- liver function
- thyroid function
- syphilis serology
- vitamin B_{12} levels
- folate levels
- bone profile
- lipid profile
- glucose
- neuroimaging – computed tomography (CT) or magnetic resonance imaging (MRI).

Electrocardiography (ECG) or chest x-ray should be carried out as determined by the clinical presentation.

Neuroimaging

In clinical practice, the two main types of neurological imaging currently used are CT and MRI.

The primary indication of CT brain scans is the exclusion of focal and/or treatable lesions, such as brain tumours, subdural and subarachnoid haemorrhages and hydrocephalus. These pathologies are found in less than 1% of cases. CT and MRI brain scans also provide information on cerebral atrophy. In older individuals, the finding of cerebral atrophy has less clinical significance, as it may be in tune with the ageing process. However, the presence of diffuse atrophy in a younger brain is more likely to be of pathological significance.

Structural neuroimaging should be carried out in all patients presenting with a young-onset dementia, to exclude other pathologies and to help establish the subtype of dementia. MRI is often preferable, as CT may not demonstrate focal atrophy well.

Functional imaging may also be helpful as it can detect focal brain dysfunction. Hexamethylpropyleneamine oxime (HMPAO) single photon emission computed tomography (SPECT) can help to differentiate the subtype of dementia. Dopaminergic iodine-123-

radiolabelled SPECT can be used to confirm suspected dementia with Lewy bodies.

Causes of early-onset dementias

The clinical presentations of the following diseases are not usually markedly different between older and younger patient groups.

Alzheimer's disease

Alzheimer's disease accounts for almost one-third of the cases of dementia in younger people. There is some evidence in younger-onset Alzheimer's disease that the symptoms of parietal lobe dysfunction are more marked. The typical presentation of Alzheimer's disease includes a progressive episodic (day-to-day) memory loss and visuospatial and perceptual deficits with well-preserved language and social functioning. In familial forms of Alzheimer's disease, decline in verbal memory and performance IQ can be the earliest signs of the disease.

Alzheimer's disease is more common in females than males. It shows increasing prevalence with increasing age. The average duration of illness is 8 years.

The preferred diagnostic criteria for Alzheimer's disease are the National Institute of Neurological and Communication Disorders and Stroke/Alzheimer's Disease and Related Disorders Association (NINCDS/ADRDA) criteria (Box 3.1).[8]

Neuroimaging in Alzheimer's disease

Structural imaging with CT or MRI may show early atrophy of the anterior temporal lobes, particularly in the dominant hemisphere,

---

Box 3.1 NINCDS/ADRDA criteria for the clinical diagnosis of probable Alzheimer's disease[8]

● Dementia established by clinical examination and documented by the MMSE, Blessed Dementia Scale, or some similar examination, and confirmed by neuropsychological tests
● Deficits in two or more areas of cognition
● Progressive worsening of memory and other cognitive functions
● No disturbance of consciousness
● Onset between the ages of 40 and 90 years most often after 65 years
● Absence of systemic disorders or other brain diseases that in and of themselves could account for the progressive deficits in memory and cognition

progressing to the parietal lobes and finally the frontal lobes as the disease progresses.

Genetics of Alzheimer's disease

Alzheimer's disease mostly occurs as a sporadic disorder, even in the younger population. However, inherited forms are more likely in the younger population. Familial Alzheimer's disease is rare, accounting for less than 10% of cases of Alzheimer's disease. Cases of familial Alzheimer's disease tend to have an early onset. Inheritance is autosomal dominant. There are many reported genetic mutations, but the three most common mutations are of the presenilin 1 gene on chromosome 14, the B amyloid precursor protein on chromosome 21 and the presenilin 2 gene on chromosome 1.[9]

Vascular dementia

Vascular dementia is the second most common cause of dementia in younger and older populations. Diagnosis is based on the clinical picture, identification of risk factors and brain imaging. The clinical presentation is variable and depends on the site and extent of the lesion.

The preferred diagnostic criteria for vascular dementia are the National Institute for Neurological Disorders and Stroke–Association Internationale pour la Recherché et l'Enseignment en Neurosciences (NINDS-AIREN) criteria.[10] These criteria state that for a clinical diagnosis of probable vascular dementia, the presentation must include all of the following:

1. the presence of dementia
2. the presence of cerebrovascular disease
3. a relationship between the above two disorders.

Syndromes of vascular dementia

1. Multiple cortical infarcts leading to a stepwise deterioration of cognitive functions
2. Small vessel disease leading to a more insidious decline of cognitive functioning
3. Strategic infarcts – small cryptic strokes that cause cognitive impairment
4. CADASIL (cerebral autosomal dominant arteriopathy with subcortical infarcts and leukoencephalopathy)

CADASIL is an uncommon cause of young-onset subcortical strokes and dementia that is caused by mutations of the Notch 3 gene on chromosome 19. MRI (Figure 3.4) typically reveals diffuse white-matter lesions of the cerebral hemispheres, especially the anterior temporal lobes and external capsules. Electron microscopy of skin biopsies may reveal characteristic granular osmophilic material.

Mixed dementia

Autopsy data suggest a high co-occurrence of Alzheimer's and vascular pathologies in individuals with dementia. Forty-eight per cent of people with Alzheimer's disease have significant cerebrovascular changes at postmortem, whilst this is the case in 33% of age-matched controls.[11] Pathology of the Alzheimer's type is found in 77% of individuals diagnosed with cerebrovascular disease.[12]

The presence of cerebrovascular disease in Alzheimer's disease patients increases the risk of developing clinical dementia. Hypertension, smoking, diabetes, age, total cholesterol, atrial fibrillation and ischaemic heart disease are well known as vascular risk factors. They are all also independent risk factors for Alzheimer's disease.

Frontotemporal cortical neurodegenerations

Frontotemporal lobar degenerations are a series of primary conditions affecting younger adult males more frequently than females. They include frontotemporal dementia (FTD), semantic dementia, primary progressive non-fluent aphasia, frontal dementia (motor neurone disease – MND), multisystem atrophy, corticobasal degeneration,

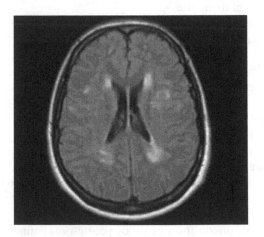

Figure 3.4   MRI scan of CADASIL

Parkinson's disease, progressive supranuclear palsy (Steele–Richardson–Olszewski) and neurofilament inclusion body disease. The average age at onset is 45 to 65 years, and the average duration of illness is 8 years. There is a positive family history in up to 50% of patients.[13]

There is an association between frontal dementia and MND. The rate of dementia in MND is much higher than expected, and indeed a significant minority of patients with FTD develop features of MND. Up to 10% of patients with MND show features of dementia. These patients usually have an aggressive course of illness.

Frontotemporal dementia

Frontotemporal dementias present in varied forms according to the area of degeneration and the differing pathologies.

From the viewpoint of behavioural neuropsychology, we recognise

(a) behavioural forms (frontal variant FTD)
(b) language forms (semantic dementias and primary progressive non-fluent aphasia) (Figure 3.5).

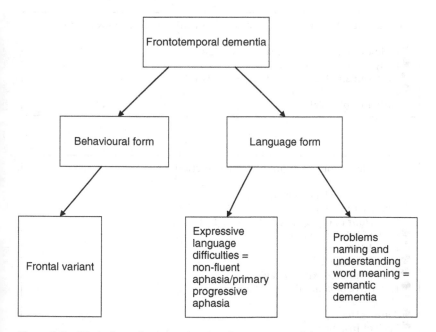

Figure 3.5 Clinical syndromes related to frontotemporal dementia

In the frontal variant, there are patchy deficits in episodic memory, perseveration, motor dysphasia, echolalia and echopraxia. In the early stages of the disease, memory and visuospatial skills are preserved. The striking clinical hallmark is the range of behavioural alterations and personality changes usually defined as 'frontal lobe syndrome' (Box 3.2). There is progressive loss of awareness of social cues, and judgement, social conduct and integration are all affected. The individual may present with varying and increasing degrees of extremes of personality, with impulsivity, disinhibition, apathy and euphoria. Features of environmental dependency, magnetism and utilisation behaviour may appear. Symptoms of frontal lobe dysfunction are given in Box 3.3

In semantic dementia, there is marked impairment of language at outset, with paraphasias, reduced fluency and poor word comprehension. Initially there is relative preservation of other cognitive domains, and tests of attention and executive functions are often initially normal. Behavioural difficulties and impairment of other cognitive domains may emerge as the disease progresses. Radiologically, the structural neuroimaging shows discrete anterior left temporal atrophy.

Box 3.2   NINDS criteria for frontal lobe dementia – core diagnostic criteria[14]

● Insidious onset and gradual progression
● Early decline in social conduct
● Early impaired regulation of personal conduct
● Early emotional blunting
● Early loss of insight

Box 3.3   Symptoms of frontal lobe dysfunction

● Change in social conduct
● Change in behaviour
● Behaviour inappropriate to the social situation
● Lack of inhibitions
● Impulsivity
● Poor judgement
● Inappropriate sexual behaviour
● Repetitive or compulsive behaviours
● Hyperorality
● Self-neglect
● Lack of insight

In primary progressive non-fluent aphasia, patients typically have a progressive decline in their language with a relative sparing of other cognitive domains. Speech is non-fluent and effortful. Speech output becomes progressively more difficult, and in the later stages the patient may become mute. Behavioural changes may occur later in the disease. Predominant atrophy of the left perisylvian fissure is seen on neuroimaging.

In the later stages of both semantic dementia and primary progressive non-fluent aphasia, the language impairment usually progresses to a complete aphasia.

Neuroimaging in frontotemporal dementia

Structural imaging with CT or MRI may show atrophy of the frontal lobes and anterior temporal lobes. Functional imaging with SPECT or positron emission tomography (PET) will typically show decreased perfusion in the frontal lobes and temporal lobes. The findings can sometimes be asymmetrical.

Dementia with Lewy bodies

The core features of dementia with Lewy bodies are progressive cognitive decline, fluctuating cognition, the presence of parkinsonian symptoms and visual hallucinations that are typically recurrent, well formed and detailed. Other features that are highly suggestive of dementia with Lewy bodies include; rapid eye movement (REM) sleep behaviour disorder (Box 3.4), severe neuroleptic sensitivity and low dopamine transporter uptake in the basal ganglia, demonstrated by SPECT or PET imaging.[15]

Dementia with Lewy bodies should be diagnosed when dementia occurs before, or concurrently with, parkinsonism. Dementia that occurs in the context of well-established Parkinson's disease is best described as Parkinson's disease dementia.

Patients who have dementia with Lewy bodies are extremely sensitive to the side effects of typical and atypical antipsychotics. Approximately

---

Box 3.4 Rapid eye movement sleep behaviour disorder (RBD)

RBD is a sleep disturbance found in Parkinson's disease. It presents with symptoms of acute motor restlessness during REM phases of sleep. In some cases, RBD occurs before the patient develops the motor symptoms of Parkinson's disease.

50% of patients with dementia with Lewy bodies will have an adverse reaction to the administration of neuroleptics.

Alcohol-related dementia

Alcohol-related dementia is a persistent dementia that occurs within the context of significant alcohol use and is not attributable to any other condition. Cognition may slowly improve if abstinence is achieved.

Heavy, prolonged alcohol use can cause damage to the limbic structures and the frontal lobes, leading to memory and executive impairments. Autobiographical memory is often affected and confabulation can occur. The memory loss is often static, although it may improve following a period of abstinence.

The radiological findings in the brains of individuals with alcohol-related dementia usually confirm the presence of atrophy, with a predilection for the superior frontal cortex. There can be also periventricular and white-matter changes. Atrophy of the cerebellar vermis is noted in severe cases.

Wernicke–Korsakoff syndrome is caused by thiamine depletion. It is distinguished by the classic triad of eye signs (ocular palsies, most likely of cranial nerve VI, with or without nystagmus), ataxia and cognitive impairment. These signs have a very high specificity, but a low sensitivity. Given this, and the variable course, the low risks of parenteral vitamin B and the potential recovery that can be achieved with effective treatment, it is important that the patient is treated aggressively and as soon as possible.

Huntington's disease

The characteristic triad of clinical features present in Huntington's disease are motor disorder, cognitive disorder and emotional disorder. However, there is variation between patients in the time of onset, specific symptoms and the progression of illness.

The characteristic motor symptom is chorea. However, dystonia, athetosis, motor restlessness, myoclonus and voluntary movement disorders may also be present. Depression, apathy and disinhibition are common neuropsychiatric symptoms and may predate the movement disorder. The cognitive domains characteristically affected in Huntington's disease include executive functioning, language, visuospatial skills and memory. The cognitive deficits can appear early in the disease and may also predate the movement disorder.

Huntington's disease is caused by expansion of the CAG trinucleotide repeat. The Huntington's disease gene is autosomal dominant and is transmitted with complete penetrance. The number of CAG repeats in normal chromosomes ranges from 11 to 34. The number of repeats required for a person to manifest the disease is 36–38. Increased numbers of CAG repeats are associated with an earlier age of onset and a greater severity of brain pathology. However, no relationship has been consistently found between increased numbers of CAG repeats and disease progression, symptoms at onset or psychiatric symptoms. Diagnostic and predictive testing is available.

Onset is generally in middle life, often in the fifth and sixth decades. The length of the trinucleotide repeats accounts for some of the variation in age of disease onset. In some families there is 'anticipation', with the disease onset occurring earlier and with greater severity in successive generations. However, in the majority of families the age of onset from generation to generation remains pretty constant. The typical duration of illness is 15 to 20 years.

Structural neuroimaging shows bilateral atrophy of the head of the caudate nucleus and atrophy of the putamen and globus pallidus. SPECT scans show cerebral hypoperfusion in the basal ganglia even before atrophy is evident on MRI scan.

Postmortem studies of the brains of patients with Huntington's disease show atrophy of the frontal lobes, caudate nucleus, putamen and globus pallidus and enlarged ventricles.

Prion diseases

Creutzfeldt–Jakob disease (CJD) tends to occur in middle life. It is rapidly progressive and often fatal in 6 months. Prodromal insomnia, malaise and depression are common. Myoclonus becomes prominent as the disease progresses. Additional symptoms include: seizures, cerebellar ataxia, cortical blindness and extrapyramidal signs. The electroencephalogram (EEG) is grossly disturbed and shows characteristic periodic triphasic wave complexes. CT imaging is often normal or may show non-specific atrophy. MRI may show high signal changes in the putamen and caudate head and cortical hypersensitivity on fluid attenuated inversion recovery (FLAIR) sequences

New variant Creutzfeldt–Jakob disease (vCJD) commonly affects younger people. The average age of onset is 26 years and the average duration of illness is 13 months. The earliest symptoms are often psychiatric and include depression, anxiety and agitation. There are no distinctive changes on EEG. MRI shows increased signal in the pulvinar. Prion protein immunostaining is positive in lymphoid tissues and therefore the diagnosis can be made from a tonsillar biopsy.

Management of younger people with dementias

The ongoing support and management of people with young-onset dementias is complex and requires input from a multidisciplinary team. However, there are few specific services for people with young-onset dementias. There is also limited awareness and understanding of people who develop dementia at an early age, thus making it difficult for patients and their carers to access support.

We have already outlined the differing needs of younger people with dementia compared to older people with dementia. General dementia services are often inappropriate for use by younger people and may not be able to meet their different needs. Age can often be a barrier to accessing services, so in some parts younger people may not even be eligible for input from general dementia services. Obviously the best solution is for services to be flexible; it may be that some people over the age of 65 years would be best suited to services for younger people with dementia, whereas some people under the age of 65 years may be better catered for by the general dementia services.

Ideally, services for younger people with dementia should be jointly commissioned by both health and social care, and have the involvement of the voluntary sector.

Non-pharmacological management strategies such as mental exercise, physiotherapy and dietary treatment, together with drug therapies may be beneficial in reducing the impact or slowing down the progression of the disease. Medications such as antipsychotic drugs may be needed for delusions and hallucinations, and serious distress or danger from behaviour disturbance. Support packages need to include appropriate day care, respite care and intensive home care as required. Support for families and carers is also required, especially in cases where there may be dependents such as children.

Pharmacological management strategies

It is important to treat any comorbid medical or psychiatric illnesses. The underlying degenerative disorder should also be treated if appropriate. Vascular risk factors should be addressed. Antidementia agents are summarised in Table 3.3.

Antidementia agents

The acetylcholinesterase inhibitors

The cholinergic hypothesis suggests that a selective loss of cholinergic neurones in Alzheimer's disease leads to reduced levels of acetylcholine

Table 3.3 Antidementia agents

Medication	Dose range	Mechanism of action	Common side effects
Donepezil (Aricept®)	5–10 mg	Acetylchoinesterase inhibitor	Nausea, diarrhoea, vomiting, anorexia
Galantamine (Reminyl®)	8–24 mg	Acetylchoinesterase inhibitor	Nausea, diarrhoea, vomiting
Rivastigmine (Exelon®)	3–12 mg	Acetylchoinesterase inhibitor	Nausea, diarrhoea, vomiting
Memantine (Ebixa®)	5–20 mg	NMDA receptor antagonist	Constipation, headache, dizziness, drowsiness

and this causes progressively deteriorating cognitive functions. There are three acetylcholinesterase inhibitors that are currently licensed for use in Alzheimer's disease for patients of any age; donepezil, rivastigmine and galantamine. The available evidence base confirms that the acetylcholinesterase inhibitors are effective across the spectrum of Alzheimer's disease (mild, moderate and severe disease) and they also lead to improvements in non-cognitive symptoms. Benefits are shown against placebo. Results of trials in other types of dementia (vascular dementia, dementia with Lewy bodies and Parkinson's disease dementia) are also positive, but the acetylcholinesterase inhibitors are not currently licensed for treatment of these conditions[16].

The acetylcholinesterase inhibitors should be prescribed with caution in patients with sick sinus syndrome or other supraventricular conduction abnormalities, those who have susceptibility to peptic ulcers, and in asthma or chronic obstructive pulmonary disease.

Memantine

Memantine is licensed for use in moderate to severe Alzheimer's disease. It is an N-methyl-D-aspartate (NMDA) receptor antagonist, which may reduce glutamate-mediated neuronal excitotoxicity.

The National Institute for Health and Clinical Excellence (NICE) has produced guidelines on the use of anti dementia agents.[17]

Antipsychotic agents

Symptoms that may respond to neuroleptic medication include physical aggression and psychotic symptoms. They should be used for the shortest time possible, at the lowest dose possible.

In March 2004 the Committee on Safety of Medicines (CSM) advised that neither olanzapine nor risperidone should be used for the treatment of behavioural and psychological symptoms in dementia. They reported that their use was associated with a threefold increase in stroke in people with dementia and that with olanzapine there was a twofold increase in all-cause mortality in this group of patients. Risperidone can be used for acute psychosis in dementia, but only on a short-term basis and under specialist advice. Olanzapine is not licensed for this use. The CSM also advised that history of, and risks for, cerebrovascular disease should be considered when prescribing these drugs.

Antidepressants

Depression occurs frequently in young-onset dementias. Symptoms of mood disturbance should always be asked about. Selective serotonin reuptake inhibitors (SSRIs) are used first line, due to their favourable side-effect profile and because any antidepressant with anticholinergic effects may worsen cognition.

Psychological and other non-pharmacological treatment strategies

Symptoms that may respond to non-pharmacological interventions include mild depressive symptoms, wandering and repetitive questioning. The ideal environment for someone with dementia is one that is constant, familiar and non-stressful. Box 3.5 summarises components of behavioural analysis that could be used in managing behavioural problems in patients with young-onset dementia.

Other therapies that have been shown to help in the management of behavioural and psychological symptoms in dementia include aromatherapy, music therapy, recreation and bright light.

Conclusions

Young-onset dementias are a fascinating group of disorders that present many challenges, particularly in terms of diagnosis, management and provision of suitable services. Dementia in younger people is less

---

Box 3.5 Behavioural analysis: ABC charts – 'antecedent, behaviour and consequences'

● Identify the target behaviour
● Identify the triggers to the behaviour
● Identify the events that follow the behaviour
● Set goals to modify the behaviour
● Evaluate and modify goals

common than dementia in later life and there is a wider differential diagnosis. The diagnosis and the symptoms of the conditions can have a devastating impact on patients, carers and their families.

To adequately address the needs of these patients and their carers, there needs to be cooperation and collaboration across all the relevant statutory and voluntary services. Carers regularly report that they would like to see better coordination of services, and to receive welfare advice, support and respite care. It is often unclear how services should be accessed, with subsequent delay in diagnosis, treatment and provision of appropriate support.

Key references

- Burns A, O'Brien J, Ames D. *Dementia*. London: Hodder Arnold; 2005.
- Hodges J. *Early-onset Dementia: a multidisciplinary approach*. Oxford: Oxford University Press; 2001.
- Murray M, Baldwin RC. *Younger People with Dementia: a multidisciplinary approach*. Oxford: Taylor and Francis; 2003.
- National Institute for Health and Clinical Excellence. *Dementia: supporting people with dementia and their carers in health and social care*. Clinical guideline 42. London: National Institute for Health and Clinical Excellence; 2006.

References

1. Kaiser S, Panegyres PK. The psychosocial impact of young onset dementia on spouses. *American Journal of Alzheimer's Disease and Other Dementias* 2006; 21(6): 398–402.
2. Williams T, Dearden AM, Cameron IH. From pillar to post – a study of younger people with dementia. *Psychiatric Bulletin* 2001; 25: 384–7.
3. Harvey RJ. *Young Onset Dementia: epidemiology, clinical symptoms, family burden, support and outcome*. London: Dementia Research Group; 1998.
4. Knapp M, Prince M. *Dementia UK – The Full Report*. London: Alzheimer's Society; 2007.
5. Department of Health. *Living Well with Dementia: a national dementia strategy*. London: Department of Health; 2009.
6. Folstein MF, Folstein SE, McHugh PR. (1975), 'Mini-mental state'. A practical method for grading the cognitive state of patients for the clinicians. *Journal of Psychiatric Research* 1975; 12(3): 189–98.
7. Mathuranath PS, Nestor PJ, Berrios GE, Rakowicz W, Hodges JR. A brief cognitive test battery to differentiate Alzheimer's disease and frontotemporal dementia. *Neurology* 2000; 55(11): 1613–20.
8. McKhann G, Drachman D, Folstein M et al. Clinical diagnosis of Alzheimer's disease: report of the NINCDS-ADRDA Work Group under the auspices of Department of Health and Human Services Task Force on Alzheimer's Disease. *Neurology* 1984; 34: 939–44.
9. Schott JM, Fox NC, Rossor MN. Genetics of the dementias. *Journal of Neurology Neurosurgery and Psychiatry* 2002; 73(Suppl II): ii27–ii31.

10. Roman GC, Tatemichi TK, Erkinjuntti T et al. Vascular dementia: diagnostic criteria for research studies. Report of the NINDS-AIREN international workshop. *Neurology* 1993; 43: 250–60.
11. Jellinger KA, Mitter-Ferstl E. The impact of cerebrovascular lesions in Alzheimer disease, a comparative autopsy study. *Journal of Neurology* 2003; 250: 1050–5.
12. Barker WWW, Luis CA, Kashuba A et al. Relative frequencies of alzheimer disease, Lewy Body, Vascular and frontotemporal dementia, and hippocampal sclerosis in the State of Florida Brain Bank. *Alzheimer Disease and Associated Disorders* 2002; 16: 203–12.
13. Sampson EL, Warren JD, Rossor MN. Young onset dementia. *Postgraduate Medical Journal* 2004; 80: 125–39.
14. Neary D, Snowden JS, Gustafson L et al. Frontotemporal lobar degeneration: a consensus on clinical diagnostic criteria. *Neurology* 1998; 51: 1546–54.
15. McKhann GM, Albert MS, Grossman M, Miller B, Dickson D, Trojanowski JQ. Clinical and pathological diagnosis of frontotemporal dementia. Report of the Work Group on Frontotemporal Dementia and Pick's Disease. *Archives of Neurology* 2001; 58: 1803–1809.
16. McKeith IG, Dickson DW, Lowe J et al. Diagnosis and management of dementia with Lewy bodies: Third report of the DLB consortium. *Neurology* 2005; 65(12): 1863–72.
17. National Institute for Health and Clinical Excellence. Donepezil, galantamine, rivastigmine and memantine for the treatment of Alzheimer's disease. Technology appraisals TA217. London: National Institute for Health and Clinical Excellence; 2011.

4
Substance Misuse and Comorbid Psychiatric Disorders

Sanjoo Chengappa and Mohammed T. Abou-Saleh

Large-scale, community-based, clinical comorbidity surveys in the United States of America (USA), western Europe and Australia have provided clear evidence that persons with psychiatric disorders, particularly schizophrenia and bipolar disorders, are much more vulnerable to alcohol and drug-use disorders than those in the general population. Substances commonly misused include alcohol and cannabis. United Kingdom (UK) studies have reported that comorbidity is usually underestimated or goes unrecognised by care coordinators. Moreover, these patients spend twice as much time in hospital as those without substance misuse. Patients with co-occurring schizophrenia and alcohol or drug use have greater risk of relapse and rehospitalisation, poor compliance with treatment, higher rates of suicide and homicide, and a worse overall response to antipsychotic medication.

The scope of this chapter is to define dual diagnosis, identify meaningful subgroups and describe key aspects of their assessment and treatment, and optimal models of care including integrated service models.

Definition

'Psychiatric comorbidity' and 'dual diagnosis' are terms used broadly to define the co-occurrence of psychiatric disorder and substance use disorder. Subgroups of patients with dual diagnosis can be defined by presumed aetiological mechanisms:

1. primary psychiatric disorder with secondary substance misuse
2. substance misuse with secondary psychiatric disorder
3. psychiatric symptoms related to substance intoxication or withdrawal.

These categories are consistent with corresponding operationally defined categories in the *Diagnostic and Statistical Manual of Mental Diseases* (4th edition; DSM-IV (American Psychiatric Association, 1994), where a distinction is made between independent (primary) psychiatric comorbidity, substance-induced comorbid psychiatric disorders and symptoms from substance use or withdrawal.

Comorbidity appears to be essentially the rule rather than the exception. The differences between people with comorbidity lie in the complexity of the interaction of dual disorders, their severity, the degree of disability, and the settings in which they occur. A pragmatic two-dimensional approach was adopted by the national guidance on good practice in dual diagnosis (Figure 4.1).[1]

However, the term comorbidity is a misnomer at times, as multiple disorders frequently coexist. Antisocial personality disorder is a common third diagnosis and comorbidity can also be complicated by physical disorders consequent to chronic substance use.

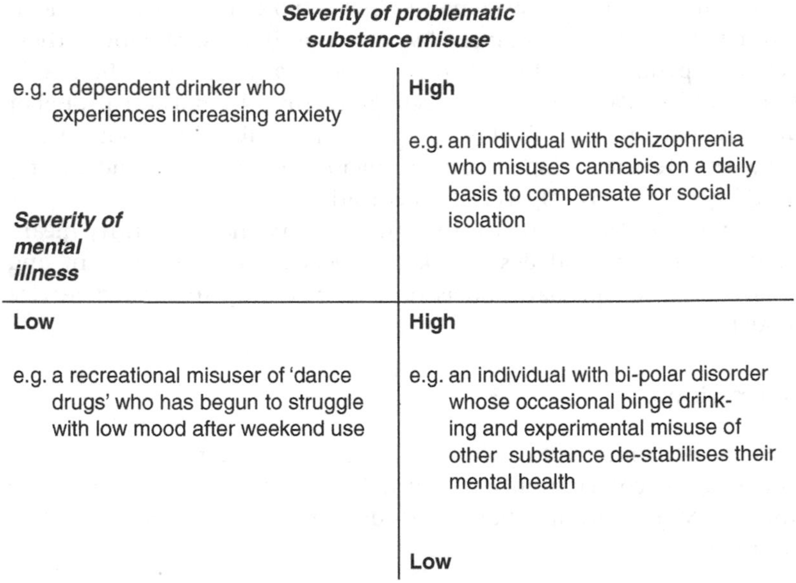

**Severity of problematic
substance misuse**

e.g. a dependent drinker who experiences increasing anxiety	**High**
	e.g. an individual with schizophrenia who misuses cannabis on a daily basis to compensate for social isolation
Severity of mental illness	
Low	**High**
e.g. a recreational misuser of 'dance drugs' who has begun to struggle with low mood after weekend use	e.g. an individual with bi-polar disorder whose occasional binge drinking and experimental misuse of other substance de-stabilises their mental health
	Low

Figure 4.1   Substance misuse and mental illness

Source: Reproduced from Department of Health. Mental Health Policy Implementation Guide: dual diagnosis good practice guide. London: Department of Health; 2002.[1]

Epidemiology

The National Comorbidity Survey, which was a national household survey from 1990 and 1992 in the USA, examined the prevalence of co-occurring mental and substance use disorder and the associations between them in the general population.[2] A total of 51.4% of the respondents in this survey with a lifetime substance use disorder also had at least one lifetime mental disorder, and 50.9% of the individuals with a lifetime mental disorder also had a history of substance use disorder. It was also observed that 42.7% of people with a 12-month substance use disorder had at least one 12-month mental disorder and 14.7% of people with a 12-month mental disorder had at least one 12-month substance use disorder.[3] The National Comorbidity Survey replication (NCS-R) followed this and was carried out between February 2001 and April 2003. A composite international diagnostic criterion was used and this showed that the lifetime prevalence of any disorder was 46.4%, and that of substance use disorders was 14.6%.[4] The 2001 National Household Survey on Drug Abuse (NHSDA) in the USA reported that in 2001 20.3% of adults with serious mental illness were dependent on or abused substances including alcohol, compared to only 6.3% of the population without a serious mental illness.[3]

European studies estimate that 60–90% of the people who misuse substances and are in treatment suffer from at least one mental health disorder and 20–50% of the people in treatment with the mental health services have a substance-related disorder, and an Australian National Survey of Mental Health and Wellbeing (NSMHW) showed that around 34% of males with an alcohol use disorder who took part in the survey also had another co-occurring psychiatric disorder.[5]

In the UK national household survey, 22% of the people with nicotine dependence, 30% of those with alcohol dependence and 45% of those with drug dependence were found to have comorbid psychiatric disorders.[6] A UK cross-sectional survey of clinical populations showed that 44% of patients with mental illness reported past-year problematic drug use and/or harmful alcohol use; 75% of drug-service and 85% of alcohol-service patients had a past-year psychiatric disorder.[7] Importantly, most of these comorbidity patients were not identified by services and received no specialist intervention.

Aetiology and risk factors

Aetiological models for comorbidity include common factor models, secondary substance misuse models, and secondary psychiatric illness models (Table 4.1). The one common factor model that is supported by evidence is the presence of antisocial personality disorder. This concurs with the clinical experience of patients with severe mental illness often having antisocial personality traits or disorder. Mueser et al., in a cohort study involving 325 patients with comorbid psychiatric disorder and substance misuse, identified that predictors of comorbidity were male gender, young age, less education, criminal activity, conduct disorder and antisocial personality disorder.[8]

Secondary substance misuse theories include both psychosocial and biological models. Under psychosocial models, self-medication, alleviation of dysphoria, multiple risk factor and supersensitivity models have been described. According to the self-medication theory, severely mentally ill patients use substances to alleviate specific symptoms or to counter the side effects of their psychotropic medications. However, there is no evidence for this from studies. The alleviation of dysphoria theory has more credence and suggests that patients with mental illness have non-specific symptoms of dysphoria and thus consume substances to ease their symptoms. The multiple risk factor model reasons that a variety of risk factors such as social isolation, poverty, lack of structured daily activity and responsibility and living in areas with increased availability of drugs are consequent to mental illness and put people at a higher risk of using drugs, leading to comorbidity. The supersentivity theory postulates that patients with severe mental illness show a higher sensitivity to the use of alcohol and substances, the use of which frequently precipitates a relapse of their illness.

Table 4.1   Dual diagnosis: a review of aetiological theories[9]

Model	Description
Common factor models	Conduct and antisocial personality disorders, low socioeconomic status, cognitive impairment

Secondary substance use disorder models	1. Psychosocial risk factor models
	   a. Self-medication
	   b. Alleviation of dysphoria
	   c. Multiple risk factor models
	2. Biological model
	3. Supersensitivity model

Secondary psychiatric disorder models	Cannabis/stimulants-induced psychosis
Bidirectional models	Substance misuse ⟷ mental illness

The secondary psychiatric illness model draws on the kindling/behavioural sensitisation hypothesis, for example cannabis use may precipitate schizophrenia or other psychotic disorders with an earlier age of onset than in those who have not used drugs.

Course and outcomes

Comorbidity of substance use disorders with mental illness leads to more severe psychiatric symptoms, greater disability, higher rates of relapse and psychiatric hospitalisation and increased use of emergency services. It is also linked to higher rates of homelessness and poor psychosocial outcomes. Comorbidity is also associated with non-compliance with medications, increased risk of blood-borne viral infections (human immunodeficiency virus [HIV], hepatitis B and C) and a higher risk for self-harm, harm to others and self-neglect.

Policy context

In the USA, the Substance Abuse and Mental Health Services Administration (SAMHSA) submitted a comprehensive *Report to Congress on the Prevention and Treatment of Co-occurring Substance Abuse Disorders and Mental Disorders* in 2002.[3] This identified a 5-year blueprint strategy where SAMHSA would lead and coordinate nationally to provide effective, capable and accountable services to prevent, diagnose and treat comorbidity. This was followed by *The President's New Freedom Commission on Mental Health* report in 2003.[10] Here the role of integrated treatments in treating co-occurring substance use and mental health disorders was clearly identified. It also stressed that though integrated treatment could be offered by one or many clinicians together, a programme or a network of services, the treatment presented should appear united and cohesive to the person receiving it.

In the UK, the National Service Framework (NSF – 1999) recognised the need to tackle comorbidity; however, it did not set standards or indicate service models to address the needs of individuals with dual diagnoses. The *Dual Diagnosis Good Practice Guide* published by the Department of Health in 2002 remedied this to some extent.[1] It noted the wide prevalence of substance use in psychiatric populations and affirmed the need for comprehensive and well-integrated care delivered by mainstream psychiatric services. The guide emphasised that integrated care is superior to care delivered in sequence by one service after another (serial care) or parallel care (services providing care concurrently) models. It also maintained that specialist drug and alcohol services would continue to provide a major contribution by way of provision of training and consultation-liaison for the majority of people with comorbidity. However, a Department of Health report in 2006 on *Dual Diagnosis in Mental Health Inpatient and Day Hospital Settings* admits that only 17% of the local implementation teams (LITs) had a plan to address dual diagnosis by the end of 2004.[11]

Assessment

The essentials of assessment include detailed assessment of the substance misuse and its interaction with psychiatric disorders; functional assessment of the impact of substance misuse on relationships, housing, work, leisure and personal goals; assessment of the risks of self-harm, harm to others, self-neglect and blood-borne viral infections; assessment of motivation for change and preferences for treatment; and treatment planning to address motivation to reduce or stop substance misuse and pressing social needs and medical and psychiatric conditions.

Assessment is based on self-report, information from informants, and laboratory tests. Optimally, diagnostic assessments should be done after completion of detoxification. This helps to clarify whether the psychiatric symptoms are a result of intoxication/withdrawal states from the substances or are induced by substances or whether there is a coexisting primary psychiatric condition. Psychiatric symptoms that last more than 4 weeks from withdrawal of the substance support a diagnosis of a primary psychiatric disorder (DSM-IV). There are a number of screening tests that could aid clinical assessment: the Dartmouth Assessment of Lifestyle Instrument; the Alcohol Use Disorders Identification Test; the Drug Abuse Screening Test; the Chemical Use, Abuse and Dependence Scale; and the Substance Abuse Treatment Scale (SATS).[12] The SATS is particularly useful for measuring treatment progress or outcomes and is also used for identifying the stage of substance misuse treatment.

Laboratory-based tests

Urine tests can identify current use of substances and hair analyses have the advantage of being able to detect substance use over longer periods of time. Breath alcohol meters and blood alcohol concentrations can be used to identify current alcohol use, and liver function tests and other biochemical tests can indicate physical sequelae related to excessive alcohol use.

Treatment challenges

Treatments available to patients with dual diagnosis vary, depending on the setting and service they present to. Various false suppositions are made of comorbidity; hence its treatment can be laden with difficulties. There is the assumption that treatment of the primary disorder, either psychiatric illness or substance use, is sufficient and the secondary disorder will resolve itself. Also there is hesitation in treating patients with psychiatric disorders who misuse substances, because of the apprehension that dangerous interactions could occur when prescribed medications are combined with substances of misuse. Another belief that results in less than effective treatment being offered is that substance misuse would undermine the treatment outcomes for comorbid psychiatric disorder. There is also an erroneous perception that treating mental disorder would reduce the motivation of the individual to address their substance use problem.

Treatment approaches

Treatment involves psychosocial and pharmacological interventions guided by a stage model of change (Box 4.1) for the most favourable selection of appropriate interventions. Psychotherapeutic treatments include a range of individual (motivational interviewing, cognitive-behavioural therapy [CBT]), group (social skills training, self-help), and family interventions. Supplementary interventions are also commonly provided, including psychopharmacological, residential and vocational rehabilitation.[13] Treatment of mental health disorders that is started during active use of substances is effective and also has some effect

---

Box 4.1 Principles of treatment of substance misuse in people with severe mental illness[14]

Assertive outreach to facilitate engagement
Close monitoring to provide structure and social reinforcement
● Integrated concurrent service
Comprehensive, wide range of interventions
Stable living situation
Flexibility and specialisation (modified approaches)
Stages of treatment: engagement, persuasion, active treatment and relapse prevention
Longitudinal perspective for relapsing and chronic disorder
Optimism – instilling hope in patients and carers

on the substance misuse itself. Interventions can be divided into bio-logical, psychological or social approaches or a combination of these, depending on the needs of the individual. The management of comorbidity is based on a comprehensive physical, psychiatric and psycho-social assessment, including assessment of risk of self-harm, harm to others, self-neglect and blood-borne infections. In general, treatment of comorbidity is guided by evidence-based principles of treatment of substance misuse in people with severe mental illness.[14]

Service models

In the UK, the USA and many other countries, mental health and addiction services have traditionally been separate, for decades. Moreover, services have separate streams of funding sometimes even competing with each other for the same public funds and resources. Also, training of their staff, their attitudes towards managing patients and eligibility criteria for entry into treatment programmes have also been different.

These historical factors have encouraged the evolution of varied models of care for people with dual diagnoses. In the serial model, serious mental illness and substance use disorder are treated sequentially by separate services. Patients are initially offered treatment by one specialist team and subsequently referred to or transferred over to the other team after treatment completion. In practice, this means that treatment for one condition is withheld until appropriate treatment is provided for the other. The condition treated first would depend on the prevailing attitudes and established policies in that care provider.

In the parallel model, patients are encouraged to obtain treatment concurrently from these independent services. Both these models put the onus on the patient to access separate services, and consequently fall short of recognising the complexities of comorbidity and the interplay between dual disorders. Patients with serious mental illness are frequently excluded from addiction services, which lack resources and training to treat them. For similar reasons, mental health services fail to detect or treat substance use disorders, resulting in poor outcomes.

In the integrated care model, the same team or service offers care for both mental health and substance use disorders. Most integrated care approaches are based on the concept of stages of treatment. This is derived from Prochaska and Diclemente's stages of change that identify distinct motivational states that patients advance through in the cycle of addictions.[15] Interventions offered at each stage should be consistent with the motivation of the individual to address their comorbid substance use disorder. Delivery of interventions in steps minimises disengagement of the patient from the services as a result of differing expectations of the patient and the clinician, and hence provides better treatment outcomes. The four different stages of treatment as identified by Osher and Kofoed are:[16]

1. *engagement* – this is a period where a trusting and therapeutic relationship is developed by regular contact with the patient
2. *persuasion* – the aim during this stage of treatment is to encourage the patient to accept that he or she has a substance use problem and to influence them to start addressing it
3. *active treatment* – begins when the patient has made some effort in trying to reduce their substance use or has managed to remain abstinent for a short period of time. The aim here is to further reduce substance use or work towards abstinence
4. *relapse prevention* – after a patient has remained free from a substance use disorder for around 6 months they are deemed to have entered this stage. Other areas such as social functioning, vocational rehabilitation, and general physical health can be looked at during this stage, with a view to helping the person integrate into the community.

Table 4.2 describes potential treatment interventions at different stages of treatment based on this model.

United Kingdom service models

In the UK, services for mental illness and substance misuse have traditionally remained separate and managing substance misuse is not seen by primary care services as a core service; hence there is a lack of resources and competencies to assess and treat comorbidity. Also there is considerable involvement of the non-statutory (voluntary) sector in providing services for people with drug and alcohol problems and these organisations are often not equipped for dealing with mental health problems.

Although the available evidence strongly supports integrated care as the optimal model of care for dual diagnosis, other working (consultation–liaison) models have been developed in the UK, for example the Kingston Community Drug and Alcohol dual diagnosis service, the Haringey Dual Diagnosis service and the Combined Psychosis and Substance Use Programme (COMPASS). All these have been cited as good practice models in the dual diagnosis guide good practice guide.[12]

Table 4.2   Treatment interventions

Potential interventions at different stages of treatment	Stage of treatment			
	Engagement	Persuasion	Active treatment	Relapse prevention
Case management	✓	✓	✓	✓
Family work	✓	✓	✓	✓
Pharmacological treatment	✓	✓	✓	✓
Assertive outreach	✓	✓	✓	
Coerced or involuntary interventions	✓	✓	✓	
Residential programmes		✓	✓	
Motivational interviewing		✓	✓	
Persuasion groups		✓	✓	
CBT counselling		✓	✓	✓
Social skills training		✓	✓	✓
Vocational rehabilitation		✓	✓	✓
Active treatment groups			✓	✓
Self-help groups			✓	✓

Source: Reproduced with permission from Noordsy DL, McQuade DV, Mueser KT. Assessment considerations. In: Graham HL, Copello A, Birchwood MJ, Mueser KT, editors. *Substance Misuse in Psychosis: approaches to treatment and service delivery.* John Wiley and Sons; 2002.[17]

Instead of having a separate caseload, the COMPASS team works on a 'hub and spoke' model of service where it supports and trains both the mental health and the substance misuse services to provide a integrated shared care approach to the patient (Figure 4.2). As part of this, the COMPASS programme developed an intensive intervention working with the assertive outreach teams and a consultation-liaison model with the other mental health teams.[18]

Service models in the United States

In the USA, there has been a significant move towards supporting integrated services for comorbid disorders. In 2005 a broad set of guidelines on treating co-occurring schizophrenia and substance use disorders to enhance existing practice was published, after a consensus conference

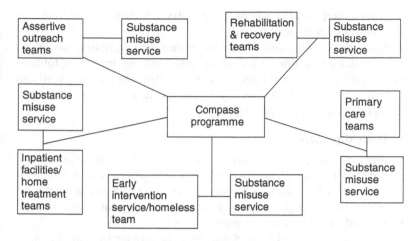

Figure 4.2 COMPASS programme

Source: Reproduced with permission from Graham HL. The combined psychosis and substance use programme: an integrated-shared care approach. In: Graham HL, editor. *Substance Misuse in Psychosis: approaches to treatment and service delivery*. John Wiley and Sons; 2003, pp. 106–20.[18]

of academic experts in the USA, which again emphasised the importance of the integrated model as the standard of care in the management of co-occurring substance use and mental health disorders.[19]

Pharmacological treatment

Substance use disorders

Pharmacological treatments are used in managing both substance use and psychiatric disorders. In substance use disorders, pharmacological treatments are mainly used to ease withdrawal symptoms during detoxification (chlordiazepoxide in alcohol detoxification) and as a substitute drug for maintenance (methadone and buprenorphine instead of heroin) in harm-reduction programmes. However, they are also used to prevent relapse by reducing craving (acamprosate in alcohol use, naltrexone in opiate use) and to treat physical consequences of substance use (for example thiamine supplements to replenish stores and carbamazepine to prevent seizures during alcohol detoxification). A wide variety of drugs are used to manage comorbid psychiatric disorders, for example antidepressants, mood stabilisers and antipsychotics. As it is beyond the scope of this chapter to describe in detail the array of drugs used in these conditions, we restrict ourselves to considering particular examples of comorbidity where specific pharmacological interventions have been shown to be of benefit.

When prescribing medications for comorbid psychiatric disorders, the potential interactions with substances of misuse, including tobacco smoking, also need to be taken into account. Patients also frequently go through unplanned discharges, and monitoring and ensuring compliance is essential to prevent relapse.

Psychotic disorders

Conventional antipsychotics are best avoided in this group because of the paucity of evidence for their effectiveness. There is also some evidence that in schizophrenia an increase in substance use is seen with the use of these drugs. Atypical antipsychotics are favoured, though further studies are required to support this.[20]

Studies have reported that clozapine is beneficial in reducing substance misuse in patients with schizophrenia. This may be mediated by improved mental state and/or side effects, or by its anti-craving effects. Individuals with alcohol use disorder co-occurring with schizophrenia or schizoaffective disorder appear to particularly benefit from the use of clozapine. Studies have shown decreases in alcohol use and increased remission of alcohol use disorders in this group.[21,22] A reduction in cannabis use in comorbid cannabis use and schizophrenia has also been noted but these results are not as robust as those seen in the alcohol use disorder group.

Mood and anxiety disorders

Symptoms of dysphoria, anxiety and depression are experienced by people with substance use disorders and these could be associated with withdrawal from drugs and alcohol. Hence, diagnosing and treating people for mood disorders should be deferred until completion of detoxification and until a period of abstinence has been achieved (3–4 weeks), unless the symptoms of the mood disorder are severe enough to necessitate immediate action.

There are not many robust studies involving antidepressants in comorbidity. One study comparing fluoxetine to a placebo group was carried out by Cornelius et al., which included people with alcohol dependence and depression, demonstrated improved outcomes for depressive symptoms with fluoxetine. Neither group remained completely abstinent during a period of 1 year; the fluoxetine group had fewer of days of drinking leading to intoxication when compared to the placebo group. However, there was no significant difference between the two groups on the total number of drinking days.[23] Existing studies suggest that specific serotonin reuptake inhibitors (SSRIs) appear to improve drinking behaviour and depressive symptoms only in severely depressed patients with alcohol dependence. Because of the potential toxic interactions between tricyclic antidepressants (TCAs) and alcohol, TCAs are best avoided in this group.

Imipramine has been shown to improve depressive symptoms in comorbid alcohol use disorders and in opiate-dependent patients receiving methadone. However, evidence for their effect on substance use is minimal. Again, due to the potential interactions, TCAs are best avoided in opiate users. SSRIs should be used with caution, as robust studies have not been carried out in this population to determine their efficacy. There is no evidence yet for the effectiveness of pharmacological treatments in cocaine users with comorbid depressive features.

Alcohol is commonly misused by people with bipolar affective disorder. Sodium valproate has shown some promise in comorbid substance use and bipolar disorders;[24] however, more research is needed in this group. Sodium valproate is also favoured over lithium because of the side effects and the serious potential interactions between drugs of misuse and lithium.

Since anxiety is a common symptom in alcohol use disorders, anxiety disorders should only be diagnosed after a period of abstinence. The British Association of Psychopharmacology suggests the use of fluoxetine as a first-line treatment and states that there is not much evidence for the use of buspirone in this group.[20]

Psychological treatments

Individual counselling interventions

Motivational interviewing/motivational enhancement therapy

Motivational interviewing has been used in the management of substance use disorders. Essentially, people modify their behaviour following awareness that their habits are preventing them from achieving their own personal goals. They are not usually motivated by the common negative consequences of substance misuse as perceived by others. Motivational interviewing works on the following principles. The therapist uses his rapport developed with the person to allow the person to identify their personal goals and recognise how substance use is interfering in the accomplishment of these goals, in a non-judgemental and non-challenging manner. When personalised feedback is added after the initial baseline assessment, to boost motivation, the extended form has been referred to as motivational enhancement therapy (MET). A modified version of this can be used to treat comorbidity.

When motivational interviewing is used in persons with comorbidity, the focus is on exploring and developing realistic personal goals, as this is crucial to overcome the disillusionment developed from the repeated disappointments and failures experienced by this group.[13]

Cognitive-behavioural therapy

Cognitive-behavioural therapy (CBT) is a structured therapy that links thoughts, emotions and behaviour and suggests that changes to one of these attributes will lead to changes in the other two. CBT has been applied in comorbidity for relapse prevention, developing social skills and gaining appropriate coping skills. These can be taught by role playing, modelling and assigning structured tasks that can be completed both inside and outside the treatment sessions.

Relapse prevention strategies target those who are currently abstinent from substances. This would include strategies to identify cues, situations and triggers that would lead a person to relapse into using substances and learning techniques to either avoid these triggers or cope with them successfully. These skills are particularly useful for persons with comorbid mental illness who use substances to cope with their feelings of dysphoria, low mood and anxiety. Coping skills to deal with cravings can also be learnt and all these can be used in the earlier stages of treatment.

Group interventions

Group approaches maybe more beneficial than individual counselling interventions, as they are based on peer support and education and include several techniques such as CBT and contingency management. They also provide a social platform for patients to support and learn from each other. As many patients can be treated at the same time, group approaches are more efficient than individual approaches.

Group work could also vary, based on the stages of treatment they target. Some of the aims of group work include supporting group members in remaining abstinent, teaching techniques to cope with cravings, and helping in developing skills managing relationships, handling conflict, interpersonal communications and anger management. Assertiveness and refusal skills enabling the person to reject substances in social situations would be valuable. Skills are taught using role-play, modelling and homework.[13] Existing research shows favourable outcomes for substance use and other related areas except outcomes for symptoms of mental illness.

Family interventions

Family interventions are used to educate, support and help families and carers develop coping skills. As significant proportions (60–80%) of people with comorbidity have some level of contact with family members, it is a common cause of tension within families. Loss of family support can lead to insecurity and homelessness that worsens the prognosis for both mental illness and substance use disorders. Frequently, individuals lose family support consequent to uncooperative, volatile and even aggressive behaviour at home. Reducing stress and anxiety for those who are either looking after or have close relationships with persons with comorbidity has been shown to improve prognosis for both mental illness and substance use disorders independently. Supporting the family in using their resources to help the person with the comorbid disorder enhances the quality of life of the patient and the family members.

In 2001, Barrowclough et al. compared an integrated treatment programme (that included motivational interviewing, CBT and family intervention) with routine care alone for people with schizophrenia and substance use disorders. This showed better outcomes in general functioning, some symptom reduction (reduction in positive symptoms) and reduction in substance use for the integrated treatment programme group.[25]

Self-help groups

People with substance use disorders often use self-help groups such as Alcoholics Anonymous and Narcotics Anonymous (NA) for support in addressing their substance misuse problems. In the USA, dual-focus self-help groups such as Double Trouble have developed, which assist people with co-occurring substance use and mental health disorders. However, because of the nature of the illness, self-help groups that include persons with comorbidity face particular difficulties. People with co-occurring mental illness can feel threatened in large groups and might be deterred from using them. Others with impaired social skills consequent to their mental illness might find these groups daunting. Some of the self-help groups are based around spiritual beliefs that could be off-putting to others who do not subscribe to these beliefs. Nevertheless, self-help groups that meet the individual needs of patients with comorbidity can be beneficial if the patient is motivated to participate in these groups.

Supplementary interventions

Case management

Case management refers to intensive multidisciplinary care offered by the team, either by assertive community treatment or otherwise as intensive case management. Though outcomes in reducing substance misuse and treating mental illness are inconsistent across studies,[26] positive results are seen in increased engagement, decreased hospitalisations and improved quality of life.

Residential rehabilitation

Residential treatments refer to supervised residential programmes in a drug-free environment and may differ from each other based on the length of these programmes (3 to 12 months). They can also vary based on the patient groups they target, the philosophy and programme of care, whether they provide care for people with drug or alcohol problems or both and whether they are gender-specific or mixed. Residential treatments that provide care for people with comorbidity provide intensive treatments in a safe environment, with support for daily living.

Long-term residential rehabilitation (more than a year) has been shown to have better substance use and other related outcomes and might also work in non-responders to other interventions.[26]

Outpatient programmes

Outpatient programmes include day programmes, day centres and evening programmes that offer various interventions for a period of time during the day. Again these differ based on the types of interventions used and the intensity and duration of the programmes.

Contingency management

Contingency management uses the principle that desired behaviours, when positively reinforced or rewarded, are likely to be repeated in the future. Target behaviours such as abstinence from drugs, clinic attendance, and compliance with medications are reinforced by material incentives when these behaviours happen, and these incentives are taken away when the target behaviours are not met. Incentives used in such programmes can be monetary incentives, amongst other things. Numerous clinical studies have noted the efficacy of contingency management in substance misuse populations, and many studies show better outcomes in people with comorbidity; however, it is still infrequently used in treatment interventions for substance use disorders and rarely in comorbidity.

Vocational rehabilitation

Residential and outpatient programmes usually provide assistance to patients in the final stages of treatment, supporting them to reintegrate into society. Participation in these programmes is shown to be of benefit as they not only provide motivation to patients to remain free from substances, but also build on patients' self-worth by helping them to contribute to society. Supported employment programmes appear to be one of the better approaches to vocational rehabilitation.

A systematic review by Drake et al. looked at various interventions used in dual diagnosis, and their effectiveness.[26] The authors concluded that group interventions, long-term residential rehabilitations and contingency management are the only interventions that show positive outcomes in this population, in relation to substance use. They also identified that other interventions showed positive outcomes in related areas of adjustment. However, the review was limited by lack of standardisation between the compared studies, the heterogeneity of the participants and interventions used amongst different studies and differing lengths of the programmes.

Conclusions

The term comorbidity or dual diagnosis was initially used broadly to signify the presence together of any mental illness and substance use disorder. Lately the term has come to refer to the co-occurrence of a severe mental illness and a substance use disorder. Comorbidity increases the rates of illness relapse, violence, rehospitalisation, homelessness and contracting blood-borne viruses such as HIV. A number of aetiological theories have been advanced but, considering the complexities of the disorders involved, one can safely reason that whatever the cause, it is likely to be heterogeneous. In the past decade much research has focused on comorbidity; nevertheless existing reviews indicate that further research is essential for establishing psychosocial and pharmacological interventions in the management of these complex disorders. Integrated treatments have the most evidence for but traditional ways of separate working and scarce resources are proving to be obstacles to putting this into practice. Attention must also be directed towards socio-environmental factors such as lack of safe housing, stigma, lack of support networks, increased availability of substances of misuse and criminalisation of people with substance use and mental disorders, all of which contribute to these disorders. These cannot be addressed only within a healthcare perspective and call for changes in public policies.

Key learning points

- There are high rates of comorbidity between substance misuse and other mental health disorders particularly in people with psychoses. The prevalence appears to be especially high in inpatient and crisis team settings, forensic settings, in inner city areas and in some ethnic groups.
- Comorbidity of substance use disorders with mental illness leads to more severe psychiatric symptoms, greater disability, poor psychosocial outcomes, non-compliance with medications, increased risk of blood-borne viral infections and a higher risk for self-harm, harm to others and self-neglect.
- Integrated care service models for people with comorbidity are more effective than serial care or parallel care models of service.
- There is evidence that psychosocial interventions e.g. motivational interviewing , group interventions, long-term residential rehabilitations and contingency management and pharmacological treatment with atypical antipsychotics are effective in this population in relation to substance use.

References

1. Department of Health. *Mental Health Policy Implementation Guide: dual diagnosis good practice guide.* London: Department of Health; 2002.
2. Kessler RC. The National Comorbidity Survey of the United States. *International Review of Psychiatry* 1994; 6(4): 365.
3. Substance Misuse and Mental Health Services Administration. Report to Congress on the Prevention and Treatment of Co-occuring Substance Abuse Disorders and mental disorders. Substance Misuse and Mental Health Services Administration; 2002.
4. Kessler RC, Berglund P, Demler O, Jin R, Merikangas KR, Walters EE. Lifetime prevalence and age-of-onset distributions of DSM-IV disorders in the National Comorbidity Survey replication. *Archives of General Psychiatry* 2005; 62(6): 593–602.
5. Abou-Saleh MT, Janca A. The epidemiology of substance misuse and comorbid psychiatric disorders. *Acta Neuropsychiatrica* 2004; 16(1): 3–8.

6. Farrell M, Howes S, Bebbington P et al. Nicotine, alcohol and drug dependence and psychiatric comorbidity: Results of a national household survey. *British Journal of Psychiatry* 2001; 179(5): 432–7.
7. Weaver T, Madden P, Charles V et al. Comorbidity of substance misuse and mental illness in community mental health and substance misuse services. *British Journal of Psychiatry* 2003; 183(4): 304–13.
8. Mueser KT, Yarnold PR, Rosenberg SD, Swett C, Miles KM, Hill D. Substance use disorder in hospitalized severely mentally ill psychiatric patients: prevalence, correlates, and subgroups. *Schizophrenia Bulletin* 2000; 26(1): 179–92.
9. Mueser KT, Drake RE, Wallach MA. Dual diagnosis: a review of etiological theories. *Addictive Behaviors* 1998; 23(6): 717–34.
10. *The President's New Freedom Commission on Mental Health: Final Report.* The President's New Freedom Commission on Mental Health; Rockville, MD: 2003.
11. Department of Health. *Dual Diagnosis in Mental Health Inpatient and Day Hospital Settings.* London: Department of Health; 2006.
12. Abou-Saleh MT. Dual diagnosis: management within a psychosocial context. *Advances in Psychiatric Treatment* 2004; 10(5): 352–60.
13. Mueser KT. Clinical interventions for severe mental illness and co-occurring substance use disorder. *Acta Neuropsychiatrica* 2004; 16(1): 26–35.
14. Drake RE, Bartels SJ, Teague GB, Noordsy DL, Clark RE. Treatment of substance abuse in severely mentally ill patients. *Journal of Nervous and Mental Disease* 1993; 181(10): 606–11.
15. Prochaska JO, Diclemente CC. *The Transtheoretical Approach: crossing traditional boundaries of therapy.* Homewood, IL: Krieger Publishing Company; 1994.
16. Osher FC, Kofoed LL. Treatment of patients with psychiatric and psychoactive substance abuse disorders. *Hospital and Community Psychiatry* 1989; 40(10): 1025–30.
17. Noordsy DL, McQuade DV, Mueser KT. Assessment considerations. In: Graham HL, Copello A, Birchwood MJ, Mueser KT, editors. *Substance Misuse in Psychosis: approaches to treatment and service delivery.* Chichester: John Wiley and Sons; 2002; Chapter 10, pp. 159–180.
18. Graham HL. The combined psychosis and substance use programme: an integrated-shared care approach. In: Graham HL et al., editor. *Substance Misuse in Psychosis: approaches to treatment and service delivery.* Chichester: John Wiley and Sons; 2002, pp. 106–20.
19. Ziedonis DM, Smelson D, Rosenthal RN et al. Improving the care of individuals with schizophrenia and substance use disorders: consensus recommendations. *Journal of Psychiatric Practice* 2005; 11(5): 315–39.
20. Lingford-Hughes AR, Welch S, Nutt DJ. Evidence-based guidelines for the pharmacological management of substance misuse, addiction and comorbidity: recommendations from the British Association for Psychopharmacology. *Journal of Psychopharmacology* 2004; 18(3): 293–335.
21. Zimmet SV, Strous RD, Burgess ES, Kohnstamm S, Green AI. Effects of clozapine on substance use in patients with schizophrenia and schizoaffective disorder: a retrospective survey. *Journal of Clinical Psychopharmacology* 2000; 20(1): 94–8.
22. Green AI, Burgess ES, Dawson R, Zimmet SV, Strous RD. Alcohol and cannabis use in schizophrenia: effects of clozapine vs. risperidone. *Schizophrenia Research* 2003; 60(1): 81–5.

23. Cornelius JR, Salloum IM, Haskett RF et al. Fluoxetine versus placebo in depressed alcoholics: a 1-year follow-up study. *Addictive Behaviors* 2000; 25(2): 307–10.
24. Hertzman M. Divalproex sodium to treat concomitant substance abuse and mood disorders. *Journal of Substance Abuse Treatment* 2000; 18(4): 371–2.
25. Barrowclough C, Haddock G, Tarrier N et al. Randomized controlled trial of motivational interviewing, cognitive behavior therapy, and family intervention for patients with comorbid schizophrenia and substance use disorders. *American Journal of Psychiatry* 2001; 158(10): 1706–13.
26. Drake RE, O'Neal EL, Wallach MA. A systematic review of psychosocial research on psychosocial interventions for people with co-occurring severe mental and substance use disorders. *Journal of Substance Abuse Treatment* 2008; 34(1): 123–38.
27. Rassool GH. *Dual Diagnosis: substance misuse and psychiatricdisorders.* Blackwell Publishing; 2002.

5
Acute and Transient Psychotic Disorders

Swaran P. Singh

> The art of classification lies in carving nature at the joints, but where mental illness is concerned, we cannot be sure that we have found the joints, or even that there are any to be found.[1]

Psychiatric literature is replete with terms for acute and transient psychotic disorders (ATPDs) such as psychogenic, reactive, hysterical, cycloid, schizophreniform, atypical and third psychosis, which share the clinical characteristics of an abrupt onset, short duration, no association with organic states and good outcome. These diagnostic labels highlight the conceptual and clinical confusion that surrounds these disorders. Reactive, psychogenic and hysterical presume aetiological distinctiveness of these conditions; cycloid and schizophreniform stress their unique clinical presentation and course; and atypical or third simply presuppose separation from the two typical disorders: schizophrenia and affective psychosis.

Many of these diagnoses maintain their regional popularity, such as reactive psychosis in Scandinavia and *bouffée délirante* in France. ATPDs are recognised in both the *International Classification of Diseases* (10th edition; ICD-10[2] and in the *Diagnostic and Statistical Manual of Mental Diseases* (4th edition; DSM-IV[3] as separate from schizophrenia and affective psychoses. However, while the ICD-10 considers *acuteness of onset* as a key, defining feature of ATPD, DSM-IV considers *duration of psychosis* of less than 6 months to be the distinguishing feature separating brief psychotic disorder and schizophreniform disorder from schizophrenia, reflecting both international consensuses on their occurrence but disagreement about their nosological status.

A number of recent publications have explored the diagnostic stability of the ICD-10 ATPD and its overlap with the historical constructs upon which the category has been based.[4-11]

Research in this area is beset with methodological challenges and shortcomings, such as inadequacies of definitions, aetiological prejudices, inadequate premorbid and follow-up assessments, and a limited understanding of the interactions between cultural influences and psychopathology.[12] Cultural factors in the presentation, course and outcome of ATPD are particularly poorly understood, despite evidence of major differences in incidence rates of ATPD between the developed and the developing world.[13] As yet, we don't know whether ATPDs actually exist in nature, whether their nosological distinctiveness can be meaningfully validated, and whether we can differentiate between subtypes of ATPD.

This chapter traces the historical evolution of different concepts of ATPD, summarises research evidence for their nosological distinctiveness and identifies gaps in the current literature. All variants of ATPD, including hysterical, reactive, psychogenic, cycloid, *bouffée délirante* and atypical psychoses have been included, except acute psychosis associated with organic conditions, substance misuse or psychoses occurring as adverse reactions of medication, postpartum psychosis and schizoaffective psychosis.

Postpartum psychosis can resemble ATPD since it can have an acute onset and a rapid remission. However, it is a gender-specific, birth-related psychotic condition, distinct from the historical and current concepts of ATPD.

The term schizoaffective psychosis was introduced by Kasanin in 1933 to represent a group of disorders with symptoms of both schizophrenia and mood disorders, with an acute onset, good premorbid functioning, and the presence of a stressful event prior to the onset of symptoms. Until around 1970, patients with such symptoms were variously classified as having atypical schizophrenia, remitting schizophrenia or cycloid psychosis.[14,15] However, the introduction of lithium and evidence of unipolar and bipolar subtypes has shifted the emphasis in schizoaffective psychosis from psychotic symptoms to mood-related symptoms.[16] Currently, in both the ICD-10 and DSM-IV, schizoaffective psychosis is defined by the presence of significant mood and psychotic symptoms but not by an acute onset or a remitting course.

ATPD: historical evolution of national traditions

The German perspective: cycloid psychosis

In 1934, Karl Kleist introduced the term *cycloid psychosis* for episodic disorders including *motility psychosis* and *confusion psychosis*, which were free of a defect state and also differed from manic-depressive disorders. Leonhard [17] added another category of *anxiety-elation psychosis*.[17] Perris derived diagnostic criteria from Leonhard's clinical descriptions,[18,19] and in a non-blind review of hospital notes, identified cycloid psychosis as a phenomenologically distinct subgroup of psychotic patients, occurring predominantly in women, with one-third experiencing a precipitating factor at the onset. Bipolarity of symptoms, a full remission and complete absence of a defect state were considered the defining features of cycloid psychosis.

In the United Kingdom (UK), two attempts were made to validate cycloid psychosis as a distinct psychotic disorder. Cutting et al. applied modified 'Perris criteria' non-blindly to the charts of over 2000 patients admitted to Maudsley Hospital over a 10-year period and found that 73 cases (3% of admissions) met this definition.[20] Ninety% of the cycloid group were women, and had prominent symptoms of perplexity, mood-incongruent delusions and hallucinations but also experienced bipolar mood swings. Brockington et al. invited Perris to examine case summaries of psychotic patients, blind to the original diagnosis.[21] Perris identified 30 cycloid patients, the majority of whom met DSM-III criteria for major affective disorder and the remainder had schizophreniform disorder or schizophrenia. Applying ICD-8 diagnostic definition, 47% of these cycloid patients would be diagnosed as having schizophrenia.

In ICD-10, cycloid psychosis is subsumed under acute and transient psychotic disorders, F23.[2,22] However Leonhard's original description of cycloid psychosis is very different from ICD-10 ATPD.[17] Not surprisingly, only half of ICD-10 ATPD cases meet Brockington's criteria for cycloid psychosis.[23] Using the DSM-III-R criteria, cycloid psychosis is assigned to a variety of diagnostic categories including schizophrenia, schizophreniform disorder, schizoaffective disorder, brief reactive psychosis, and affective psychotic disorders.[24] More recently, Peralta and Cuesta[25] applied Perris and Brockington criteria to a large cohort of psychosis patients and found that while cycloid psychosis syndrome could be differentiated from other psychotic disorders, it did not correspond to any DSM III-R, DSM-IV or ICD-10 category of psychosis. The diagnostic separation and distinctiveness of 'cycloid psychosis' has not, as yet, gained international recognition.

The Scandinavian perspective: reactive and psychogenic psychoses

Jaspers' original description of a psychological reaction (*reactivity*) included a temporal relationship between a stressor and a disorder, and a psychodynamic meaning to the disorder in the context of the stressor. August Wimmer described psychogenic psychoses as clinically distinct disorders in which a psychotic state occurred in a predisposed individual following a mental trauma;[26] the form and content of the mental state reflected the trauma; and the disorders remitted without deterioration. The concept was therefore akin to Jaspers' concept of psychological reaction, as applied to psychotic disorders with a good outcome. However, in the English-speaking world, psychogenic psychoses never really became popular because of the looseness and variations in the definition of the term, emphasised by Aubrey Lewis,[27] who recommended giving the term psychogenic 'a decent burial'.

Reactive psychoses: clinical features

Several attempts have been made to identify reactive psychosis as a clinically distinct disorder.[28-31] The most extensive and influential effort was by McCabe,[31] who described acuteness of onset following stress, affective features, non-schizoid premorbid personality, absence of autism, preservation of affect, brief duration of illness, and lack of family history of schizophrenia as typical of reactive psychoses. Some retrospective, non-blind case note reviews have confirmed a female preponderance, good long-term outcome and no change in diagnosis over 10–15 year follow-up.[30,32]

Reactive psychoses: cross-cultural data

In developed countries, reactive psychoses continue to feature in case reports,[33-36] especially in individuals in highly stressful jobs such as air force and naval aviation.[37,38] Acute reactive psychoses with paranoid symptoms are also noted frequently in immigrant groups,[39-43] and individuals exposed to war trauma.[44]

Reactive psychosis is also frequently reported from the developing world, mainly in the Indian subcontinent and Africa.[45-53] In many parts of Africa, brief reactive psychoses are among the commonest presentations in general hospitals,[51] and may represent transient psychotic episodes in culture-bound syndromes, although about one-fifth turn out to have schizophrenia on follow-up.[49,50]

The diagnostic status of reactive/psychogenic psychosis continues to be contentious. It is unclear whether the label is applied to any psychosis that is triggered by a stressful life event, or whether it describes a distinct clinical entity. While life events have been linked to the emergence of both schizophrenia and affective psychosis,[54] life event scales do not capture Jasper's original concept of reactivity. Hence, despite the intuitive elegance of psychosis being a meaningful psychological response to a stressor, the term is currently more popular in clinical use than in empirical research. The clinical concepts of psychogenic or reactive also do not lend themselves to empirical validation, especially in avowedly atheoretical diagnostic systems such as the DSM-IV and ICD-10.

The American/Indo-Asian perspective: hysterical psychosis

Hysterical psychosis was first described by Hollender and Hirsch as a sudden onset of florid psychotic symptoms, volatile mood and grossly abnormal behaviour, which follows a profoundly upsetting event, lasts between one and three weeks and occurs in women, usually with premorbid hysterical personality traits.[55] Langness refuted this formulation,[56] considering hysterical psychosis to be a form of culture-bound syndrome, best understood as learned behaviour in a particular socio-cultural milieu.

Attempts at validating Hollander and Hirsch's concept of hysterical psychosis have produced mixed results. While Gift and colleagues found that in a sample of 217 patients hospitalised for the first time with a functional psychiatric illness, none met Hollender and Hirsch's criteria,[57] Chinchilla and colleagues identified 30 cases from a Spanish psychiatric hospital's case records who fully met the criteria.[58] In the Spanish study, three-quarters of patients with hysterical psychosis were women, 70% had a stressful precipitant with an acute onset, 60% had fluctuating symptoms and 100% attained full remission (on an average within 23 days). The diagnosis was stable in 28 cases (93%) over 5 years.

Hysterical psychosis has also been reported from the developing world.[59,60] However, the underlying aetiological assumptions vary from it being a dissociative state, a culturally influenced reaction to extreme stress or a transient episode in the clinical presentation of post-traumatic stress disorder.[33,41,43,61-64]

The French perspective: *bouffée délirante*

Bouffée délirante was first described by Magnan as a psychotic state characterised by (a) a sudden onset without the presence of a stressful event, (b) florid and intense delusional thinking, (c) a rapidly changing clinical picture with clouding of consciousness, emotional instability, confusion, anxiety, agitation, impulsiveness and expansiveness, (d) absence of any organic pathology, (e) rapid and full recovery within a matter of days or weeks and (f) a tendency to recurrence.[65] In the early 1970s, *bouffée délirante* was diagnosed in about 4% of hospitalised patients in France.[66] The diagnostic category has gradually declined in popularity in France, with the diagnosis being given mainly to migrants on first admission. When reassessed using ICD criteria, *bouffée délirante* cases are reassigned a range of different diagnoses, and do not correspond to any particular ICD category.[67]

Using empirical criteria, Metzger identified over 300 cases of *bouffée délirante* (two-thirds of whom were female) from a large cohort of acute psychotic patients.[68] Over an average 6-year follow-up, 34% had only a single episode, 24% had recurrent and transient episodes, 34% developed schizophrenia and 7% developed a bipolar disorder. The absence of a life stressor prior to onset predicted chronicity or relapse. In a more recent attempt to delineate a clinically distinct group,[69] a cohort of 91 cases of '*bouffée délirante polymorphe*' was identified over 18 months in a French hospital. Most cases were rediagnosed as schizophrenia, affective psychosis or delusional disorder on follow-up.

The difference between the French and other psychiatric traditions partially stems from the fact that the French divide non-affective functional psychoses into acute (*bouffée délirante*) and chronic, and place far less emphasis on Schneiderian criteria for the diagnosis of schizophrenia.[70] *Bouffée délirante* has therefore survived in France without having been accepted internationally.

The Japanese perspective: atypical psychoses

Fukuda and Hatotani have reviewed the development of the Japanese concept of atypical psychoses.[71,72] This view emphasises the alteration of consciousness in symptomatology, a possible relationship to epilepsy as well as schizophrenia and bipolar disorders, and conceptual similarity to cycloid psychoses and *bouffée délirante*. However, there is very little published research to allow comparison of the Japanese and European constructs of ATPD.

The development of ICD-10 acute and transient psychotic disorders: the World Health Organization studies

The SCAAPS studies
The World Health Organization (WHO) carried out a collaborative study using the specially constructed 'Schedule for the Clinical Assessment of

Acute Psychotic States' (SCAAPS schedule).[73] The SCAAPS schedule was sent to 14 centres around the world and data collected on over 1000 cases. Acute psychosis cases were found to have a brief, good-outcome illness with no major gender differences and with schizophrenic symptoms common at initial presentation. Only half the sample had an immediate precipitating stressor. Using the SCAAPS schedule, Okasha and colleagues confirmed the existence of an acute, non-affective, non-schizophrenic psychosis in Egyptian patients.[74,75] The WHO took these finding into account when designing the ICD-10 category 'Acute and transient psychotic disorders' (F-23).

The DOSMED studies

Susser and colleagues[13,76,77] have extensively explored data from the Determinants of Outcome of Serious Mental Disorders Study (DOSMED)[78,79] to delineate non-affective acute remitting psychoses. In the total DOSMED sample, they identified a distinct subgroup of non-affective acute remitting psychosis that had a 1-week onset, either a single psychotic episode followed by complete remission, or two or more psychotic episodes with complete remission between all or most of the episodes.[13] The incidence rate was twice as high in women as in men, and in the developing world the overall incidence was about ten-fold greater than in the industrialised world for both sexes. DOSMED data from Chandigarh, North India also confirmed the existence of this acute brief non-affective psychosis with a benign long-term course.[76,77,80]

While national traditions have ensured the survival of different diagnostic terms for ATPD against the pressures of international psychiatric consensus, the boundaries between variants of ATPD are blurred. Some studies use the terms acute paranoid reaction, *bouffée délirante* and reactive psychosis interchangeably.[81] Others report similarities and overlap between reactive psychosis and *bouffée délirante*,[82] between reactive psychosis and cycloid psychosis,[83] between reactive psychosis and hysterical psychosis,[84] between ICD-10 ATPD and psychogenic and cycloid psychoses,[7] and between the European and Japanese concepts of atypical psychoses.[72]

Acute and transient psychosis: acuteness and transience

ATPD has an acute onset and presents with a florid psychotic state, which develops within a matter of hours or days. The entire range of psychiatric symptoms can appear in a polymorphic, rapidly changing picture, with confusion/perplexity, clouding of consciousness and affective instability. The clinical picture can vary between cultures, with more histrionic and excitement symptoms in India and Africa as compared to the west.[45,49] The two key defining features of ATPD however are an acute onset and an early remission.

Onset in ATPD

Acute onset of illness has long been considered a good prognostic indicator in schizophrenia.[85–88] The International Pilot Study of Schizophrenia showed that, compared to insidious onset, acute-onset cases had a significantly better 2-year prognosis, with no difference between the developing and the developed world.[78] Westermeyer and Harrow found that acuteness of onset was the best predictor of the absence of psychotic symptoms at follow-up, and was better than several other clinical and social demographic prognostic indicators.[89] Brief psychoses, which do not have an acute onset, show only a weak association with sex or socio-cultural setting and often evolve into chronic disorders.[77] The persistent ambiguity in the dual usage of the term 'acute', to imply both 'suddenness' of emergence and severity of psychopathology, has not been adequately addressed in research. Two recent studies have attempted to develop and validate operational criteria for onset, and a scale is now available for exploring the components and chronology of onset in psychosis.[11,90]

Transience (remission) in ATPD

In the 1930s, Gabriel Langfeldt suggested that the diagnosis of schizophrenia should be restricted to disorders with a poor long-term outcome, which would identify a homogenous group of schizophrenia and a heterogeneous group of good-outcome schizophreniform psychoses.[91,92] Schizophreniform psychosis was introduced in the DSM-III in 1980 as a schizophrenia-like illness but with a duration of less than 6 months. Langfeldt later observed that the DSM-III definition of schizophreniform disorder had 'nothing to do with the psychiatric states described in my paper'.[93] The category of schizophreniform psychosis has remained in successive editions of DSM-III-R and DSM-IV, with the only change being in the minimum duration criteria from 2 to 4 weeks and the addition of good and poor prognostic factors.

The diagnostic validity of schizophreniform psychosis remains doubtful. Some researchers have suggested that schizophreniform disorder can be distinguished from both schizophrenia and affective psychosis at initial examination.[94,95] However the predictive value of the good prognostic features of schizophreniform disorder is poor, the diagnosis is unstable over time, and its long-term outcome is somewhere between schizophrenia and affective psychoses.[91,96–100] Langfeldt's original cases of schizophreniform psychosis meet the DSM-III-R criteria mainly for affective disorders with psychotic features.[91,96,97] There are no empirical data to support any particular duration criterion of the first psychotic episode, which would identify a psychotic subgroup distinct from schizophrenia or affective psychosis, although 'transient' psychotic disorders appear to have a better outcome.[101] Keith and Mathews (1991) found that very few studies had addressed duration issues in psychosis.[102] The only conclusion that can be drawn from outcome studies of schizophrenia is that a longer duration of psychosis predicts a poorer outcome. As for brief psychotic disorders, Keith and Mathews stated that *'very few psychotic episodes last less than one month, and those that do, we know almost nothing about'*.[102] The conceptual problems of defining a psychotic disorder by duration alone is said to create a phenomenon akin to the Heisenberg's Principle of Uncertainty: *'the entity you are measuring moves simply by virtue of how you define it'*.[103]

The ICD-10 and DSM-III-R differ on how duration is conceptualised and measured. For a diagnosis of schizophrenia, the ICD-10 requires 1 month of *psychotic symptoms* and specifically excludes prodromal symptoms, the DSM-III-R criterion requires a 6-month duration of *illness*, but only 1 week of *psychotic symptoms*; the rest of the duration may constitute prodromal or residual symptoms. The DSM-IV has changed the duration criteria for a diagnosis of schizophrenia to a minimum of 1 month of psychotic symptoms, but retained 6 months of illness. It is as yet unclear whether this will improve the concordance between ATPD subgroups within the two systems. Several studies have suggested that ICD-10 duration criteria for ATPD are too restrictive.[104–106] DSM-IV criteria on the other hand may be too short for brief psychosis and too long for schizophrenia. There is also lack of clarity on the difference between remission and recovery. Recent attempts at developing criteria for remission based on symptom rating scales[107] are suitable for research purposes but clinically perhaps the distinction between remission and recovery should be based upon the latter constituting complete absence of psychopathology and full return to premorbid functioning.[11] ICD-10 and DSM-IV criteria for remitting psychotic disorders are compared in Table 5.1.

ATPD: current status

Recent studies on ICD-10 ATPD suggest that the criteria do identify a good-outcome group as compared to schizophrenia.[8,11,105,106,108,109]

Table 5.1   Comparison of remitting psychotic disorders in the ICD-10 and DSM-IV

Features	ICD-10	DSM-IV
Diagnostic categories	Acute and transient psychotic disorders F23	Brief psychotic disorder 298.8 and Schizophreniform disorder 295.4
Clinical presentation	'Polymorphic' and rapidly changing picture; subdivided into ATPD with or without symptoms of schizophrenia	No clinical distinction from schizophrenia other than duration
Key criteria		
Onset	Acute onset, within 2 weeks	Not a criterion
Duration	Less than 1 month for schizophrenia-like ATPD and less than 3 months for non-schizophrenia-like ATPD	1 day to 1 month for brief psychotic disorder; 1–6 months for schizophreniform disorder
Presence of stressor	'Acute stress' specified by fifth digit	'Marked stressor' specified by fifth digit; post-partum onset separately specified
Recovery	Complete recovery	'Full return to premorbid level of functioning', except where schizophreniform disorder has been diagnosed 'provisionally' with less than 6 months of illness

Cross-cultural differences also exist in diagnostic stability, with greater diagnostic instability in the developed world as compared to the developing world.[7,11,100,110] The value of having subgroups of ATPD has been questioned, since the small numbers virtually preclude empirical validation of individual subgroups.[11,110] There is also some concordance between ICD-10 ATPD and the historical constructs such as cycloid psychosis, *bouffée délirante*, schizoaffective psychosis and schizophreniform psychosis.[4,5,23,109] Several other studies, which have not used ICD-10 criteria, have also confirmed the occurrence of brief, remitting psychotic disorders with a distinct epidemiological profile.[105,106,110]

Modestin and colleagues found that the clinical presentations of non-affective functional psychoses at first admission do not allow prognostic long-term forecasts;[112] initial differences between individual diagnostic categories disappear over time. While the DSM-III-R, DSM-IV and

ICD-10 all have criteria for brief and acute psychotic disorders, these bear little relationship to the original concept of reactive or hysterical psychosis.[113] McGorry et al. concluded that while there is high concordance between various historical concepts of ATPD, these have a low concordance with DSM-III schizophrenia.[114] Even the high inter-rater reliability for reactive psychosis among Scandinavian psychiatrists[115] simply confirms diagnostic consensus within national traditions but does not allow international comparisons.

International diagnostic criteria, such as the ICD-10 and DSM-IV, are based on symptoms rather than any suggestive aetiology, and do not encapsulate concepts such as reactivity. The broad but non-specific therapeutic efficacy of psychiatric drugs has also not facilitated a symptom-based categorisation of psychotic disorders. This divergence of historical concepts and international criteria is likely to continue, since European psychiatrists give pre-eminence to psychopathology and formulation in individual cases, while Anglo-Saxon psychiatrists place emphasis on the quantification and reliability of diagnostic criteria.[116] ICD-10 ATPD criteria have attempted to bring together overlapping historical concepts, but in the absence of empirical evidence that might convert such constructs into diagnostic criteria, the ICD-10 has selected the two, shared aspects that lend themselves to measurement – acute onset and early remission. A recent study of an inception cohort of first-episode psychosis,[11] while confirming the occurrence of ATPD in a small subgroup, has cast doubt on whether acute onset and early remission are sufficient by themselves to identify a distinct subgroup of good-outcome cases. Good outcome in this study was associated with female gender and good premorbid functioning rather than with acute onset or early remission of the first psychotic episode. However, other studies using longer-duration criteria than those stipulated in the ICD-10 confirm that acute-onset, non-affective remitting psychotic disorders are a highly distinctive group, even in the industrialised world.[105,111]

Is ATPD a 'third' psychosis?

The nosological distinctiveness of ATPD is intimately linked with the categorisation of psychotic disorders *per se*. ATPD is diagnosed once schizophrenia and affective psychosis have been excluded. This presumes that both schizophrenia and affective psychosis are unitary concepts, with sharp demarcations, which would facilitate the identification of a 'third', non-affective, non-schizophrenic psychosis. The heterogeneity in the current diagnostic constructs of schizophrenia and affective psychosis has been well documented.[117-119] McGorry et al. have argued that the introduction of operationally defined diagnoses has led to 'spurious precision' and that considerable misclassification of psychotic disorders occurs from variability in the method of assigning the diagnostic criteria, rather than the criteria themselves.[117] Even small differences in the operational criteria for psychotic disorders lead to considerable inconsistencies in diagnoses.[120] Therefore, the availability of reliable operational criteria is a necessary, but not a sufficient condition for establishing the nosological distinctiveness of a disorder.

Even the 'precise' application of diagnostic criteria to clinical information does not reduce the overlap between categories of psychotic disorders. The 'atheoretical' approach to diagnosing schizophrenia, underlying current international systems, is based primarily upon the presence of Schneiderian first-rank symptoms, which have high sensitivity but low specificity and poor prognostic significance.[121,122] There is considerable overlap between schizophrenia and affective psychosis, especially when they are distinguished solely on the basis of signs and symptoms. Affective psychosis too is a heterogeneous group, comprising unipolar psychotic depression, bipolar psychotic depression and psychotic mania. Many studies have reported continuity between the two disorders, which suggests an underlying dimension of a psychotic process.[123-126] The validation of the nosological status of ATPD is therefore partly dependent upon clearer demarcation of the boundaries of schizophrenia and affective psychosis. Munro holds the contrary view, suggesting that the lack of recognition of intermediate disorders prevents a clearer demarcation between schizophrenia and affective psychosis.[127] Either way, the nosological distinctiveness of any one functional psychosis is contingent upon clearer boundaries of the rest.

Categories and dimensions of psychotic disorders

In a latent class analysis of first-episode schizophrenia patients, Castle et al. distinguished three latent classes: a neurodevelopmental type (predominantly male), a schizoaffective type (almost entirely female) and a paranoid type (with equal sex ratio).[128] The schizoaffective type was characterised by affective symptoms, a family history of affective psychosis rather than schizophrenia, better premorbid functioning and a relapsing and remitting course. This description is strikingly similar to our ICD-10 ATPD group. In their latent class analysis of the Roscommon study cohort, Kendler and Walsh proposed that there are six discrete categories of psychosis, which bear 'substantial resemblance to current or historical nosologic constructs'.[129] Several recent studies have explored the dimensions of psychopathology in psychotic disorders.[130,131] The 'negative dimension', with an insidious onset and affective flattening, has been consistently found to be associated with poor outcome.[130,132,133] The association between insidious onset and male gender [132] may partly explain the association between an acute onset, female gender and good outcome in ATPD.[134]

Should ATPD be abandoned as a diagnostic category?

Given the heterogeneity across all psychotic disorders, should one abandon the search for a new category of non-affective, non-schizophrenic psychosis? There are at least three arguments for keeping ATPD as a distinct category. The first is the clinical utility of recognising a good-outcome group in first-episode psychosis and the associated advantages in predicting the course and devising long-term treatment strategies. Patients with ATPD present such a vivid contrast to those with a chronic or deteriorating course that it is reasonable to maintain a category that signals this contrast. Secondly, and perhaps more importantly, the significant cross-cultural differences in the incidence rates of ATPD and the outcome of psychosis cannot easily be discounted.[13,79] These differences may reflect differences in exposure to 'psychogenic' stressful events in different populations, transient organic conditions, cultural differences in the experience and expression of distress, the ability to seek help and the availability of such help. Fisch reported a link between marriage and emerging psychosis in an orthodox Jewish community in Jerusalem,[135] highlighting the influence of traditional belief systems in shaping the experience of stress. In India, new 'categories' of acute psychotic states continue to appear, such as 'the Gulf bride syndrome', a sudden-onset florid agitated state with disorganised behaviour and rapidly changing clinical picture among young women who emigrate to the Gulf states soon after marriage (Professor SD Sharma, personal communication). Mezzisch and Lin have argued that the whole group of culture-bound syndromes should be classified as acute and transient psychotic disorders.[136] Thirdly, psychiatric nosology is based on research primarily conducted in the developed world but if our classification systems are designed to be truly global, research effort should be tailored to areas such as ATPD and conducted in the developing world. As economic development in countries such as India and China translates into increased research capacity, current nosological certainties may be significantly challenged, and maintaining categories that will facilitate such research is vital, especially in areas of genetics and biology.

Could ATPD in the developing world be a variant of affective disorders? There are very few published data on cultural differences in the epidemiology and outcome of affective disorders. We do not know whether the excess of ATPD in a population group is associated with fewer diagnoses of affective psychosis. Culture-specific symptoms can lead to misidentification of both mania and depression.[137,138] However epidemiological data, which would allow comparison of diagnostic traditions in the developing world, are not currently available. Further cross-cultural research may shed light on the reasons behind cultural differences in the rates of ATPD; in the meantime, it is important to ensure that international classification systems reflect international variations in psychiatric disorders.

Future implications

It has already been recommended that the ICD-11 and DSM-V should have a specific category of ATPD.[11,76,104,106] However, a specific criterion-based definition of onset should be included to improve the precision of operational criteria for ATPD. Onset in psychosis is not only poorly researched, it is also poorly conceptualised. There has been practically no research into the chronology and components of the onset of psychosis, and some of the uncertainty probably resides in the nebulous nature of the phenomenon itself. However, if onset is to be a diagnostic criterion, it needs a clearer definition, and some empirical validation of the time period of onset. We propose that a specific criterion-based definition of onset be included: onset is the time between the first reported/observed change in mental state/behaviour and the development of psychotic symptoms. Such a definition has been used in one study of ATPD.[11] This definition includes both the beginning of onset, i.e. first change, including prodromal symptoms; and its termination, i.e. onset ends when any psychotic symptoms emerge and reach a diagnostic threshold. Such a construct of onset has been used in an onset scale, which appears to identify reliably such changes in emerging psychosis.

Secondly, the relationship between stress and psychosis is still poorly understood. Identifying a group of psychotic disorders that are precipitated by stress and have a good outcome, would enhance our understanding of the biological and psychosocial variables that influence the course and outcome of psychosis. In the stress-vulnerability paradigm of psychosis aetiology, much research effort has been focussed on the 'vulnerability' such as genetics and neurodevelopmental insults, and relatively little on stress and life events. Many current controversies, such as the excess of schizophrenia in immigrant groups, the role of psychological versus pharmacological treatments and early detection and intervention in high-risk groups might be illuminated by a greater understanding of the relationship between stressful life events and psychotic disorders.

Key learning points

● Acute and transient psychotic disorders (ATPDs), which are distinct from both schizophrenia and bipolar disorders, are reported worldwide and have an interesting epidemiological profile, with an excess in women and in the developing world.

● ATPDs have traditionally been described according to the perceived uniqueness of their psychopathology (atypical psychoses/*bouffée délirante*), aetiology (reactive/psychogenic/hysterical), or course (cycloid psychosis). There are few studies on the biology, family history, premorbid characteristics or outcome of these disorders.

● The relationship between ATPD and stressful life events, their course and outcome, and the influence of culture on psychopathology remain unanswered questions requiring further research.

References

1. Kendell RE. Diagnosis and classification. In: Kendell RE, Zealley AK, editors. *Companion to Psychiatric Studies.* Edinburgh: Churchill Livingstone; 1983, p. 221.
2. World Health Organization. *The ICD-10 Classification of Mental and Behavioural Disorders: clinical descriptions and diagnostic guidelines.* Geneva: World Health Organization; 1992.
3. American Psychiatric Association. *Diagnostic and Statistical Manual of Mental Disorders.* IV edition. Washington, DC: American Psychiatric Association; 1994.
4. Marneros A, Pillmann F, Haring A, Balzuweit S, Bloink R. The relation of 'acute and transient psychotic disorder' (ICD-10 F23) to bipolar schizoaffective disorder. *Journal of Psychiatric Research* 2002; 36(3): 165–71.
5. Pillmann F, Haring A, Balzuweit S, Bloink R, Marneros A. Bouffee delirante and ICD-10 acute and transient psychoses: a comparative study. *Australia and New Zealand Journal of Psychiatry* 2003; 37(3): 327–33.
6. Pillmann F, Haring A, Balzuweit S, Bloink R, Marneros A. The concordance of ICD-10 acute and transient psychosis and DSM-IV brief psychotic disorder. *Psychological Medicine* 2002; 32(3): 525–33.

7. Sajith SG, Chandrasekaran R, Sadanandan Unni KE, Sahai A. Acute polymorphic psychotic disorder: diagnostic stability over 3 years. *Acta Psychiatrica Scandinavica* 2002; 105(2): 104–109.
8. Jager MDM, Hintermayr M, Bottlender R, Strauss A, Moller HJ. Course and outcome of first-admitted patients with acute and transient psychotic disorders (ICD-10:F23). Focus on relapses and social adjustment. *European Archives of Psychiatry and Clinical Neuroscience* 2003; 253(4): 209–15.
9. Castagnini A, Bertelsen A, Munk-Jorgensen P, Berrios GE. The relationship of reactive psychosis and ICD-10 acute and transient psychotic disorders: evidence from a case register-based comparison. *Psychopathology* 2007; 40(1): 47–53.
10. Marneros M, Pillman F. *Acute and Transient Psychoses*. Cambridge: Cambridge University Press; 2004.
11. Singh SP, Burns T, Amin S, Jones PB, Harrison G. Acute and transient psychotic disorders: precursors. Acute and transient psychotic disorders: precursors, epidemiology, course and outcome. *British Journal of Psychiatry* 2004; 185: 452–9.
12. Manschreck TC, Petri M. The atypical psychoses. *Culture Medicine and Psychiatry* 1978; 2(3): 233–68.
13. Susser E, Wanderling J. Epidemiology of nonaffective acute remitting psychosis vs schizophrenia. Sex and sociocultural setting. *Archives of General Psychiatry* 1994; 51(4): 294–301.
14. Zaudig M. Cycloid psychoses and schizoaffective psychoses – a comparison of different diagnostic classification systems and criteria. *Psychopathology* 1990; 23(4–6): 233–42.
15. Lapensee MA. A review of schizoaffective disorder: I. Current concepts. *Canadian Journal of Psychiatry* 1992; 37(5): 335–46.
16. Marneros A. The schizoaffective phenomenon: the state of the art. *Acta Psychiatrica Scandinavica Supplement* 2003; 418: 29–33.
17. Leonhard K. [Prognostic diagnosis of endogenous psychoses with reference to cycloid psychoses]. *Wiener Zeitschrift für Nervenheilkunde und deren Grenzgebiete* 1967; 24(4): 282–96.
18. Perris C. A study of cycloid psychoses. *Acta Psychiatrica Scandinavica Supplement* 1974 ; 253: 1–77.
19. Perris C, Eisemann M [Cycloid psychoses and their status within the scope of the classification of endogenous psychoses]. *Psychiatrie, Neurologie und Medizinische Psychologie. Beihefte* 1986; 33: 48–53.
20. Cutting JC, Clare AW, Mann AH. Cycloid psychosis: an investigation of the diagnostic concept. *Psychological Medicine* 1978; 8(4): 637–48.
21. Brockington IF, Perris C, Kendell RE, Hillier VE, Wainwright S. The course and outcome of cycloid psychosis. *Psychological Medicine* 1982; 12(1): 97–105.
22. World Health Organization. *The ICD-10 Classification of Mental and Behavioural Disorders – Diagnostic Criteria for Research DCR-10*. Geneva: World Health Organization; 1994.
23. Illmann F, Haring A, Balzuweit S, Bloink R, Marneros A.Concordance of acute and transient psychoses and cycloid psychoses. *Psychopathology* 2001; 34(6): 305–11.

24. Franzek E, Becker T, Hofmann E, Flohl W, Stober G, Beckmann H. Is computerized tomography ventricular abnormality related to cycloid psychosis? *Biological Psychiatry* 1996; 40(12): 1255–66.
25. Peralta V, Cuesta MJ. Cycloid psychosis: a clinical and nosological study. *Psychological Medicine* 2003; 33(3): 443–53.
26. Wimmer A. *Psykogene Sindssygdomsformer.* Copenhagen: Gad, St Hans Hospital, Jubilee Publication; 1916.
27. Lewis A. 'Psychogenic': a word and its mutations. *Psychological Medicine* 1972; 2: 209–15.
28. McCabe MS. Reactive psychoses, a clinical and genetic investigation. *Acta Psychiatrica Scandinavica Supplement* 1975; 259: 1–133.
29. McCabe MS. Symptom differences in reactive psychoses and schizophrenia with poor prognosis. *Comprehensive Psychiatry* 1976; 17(2): 301–307.
30. Andersen J, Laerum H. Psychogenic psychoses. A retrospective study with special reference to clinical course and prognosis. *Acta Psychiatrica Scandinavica* 1980; 62(4): 331–42.
31. Munoz RA, Amado H, Hyatt S. Brief reactive psychosis. *Journal of Clinical Psychiatry* 1987; 48(8): 324–7.
32. Vicente N, Ochoa E, Rios B. Psychogenic paranoid psychosis: an empirical study. *European Psychiatry* 1996; 11: 180–4.
33. Johnson LB, Proskauer S. Hysterical psychosis in a prepubescent Navajo girl. *Journal of the American Academy of Child Psychiatry* 1974; 13(1): 1–19.
34. Phelan D, Daly RJ. Koro-like syndrome associated with brief reactive psychosis in an Irish male. *Irish Medical Journal* 1996; 89(2): 75–6.
35. Ungvari GS, Hantz PM. Reactive psychosis among elderly people. *Acta Psychiatrica Scandinavica* 1990; 82(2): 141–4.
36. Ungvari GS, Leung HC, Tang WK. Reactive psychosis: a classical category nearing extinction? *Psychiatry and Clinical Neuroscience* 2000; 54(6): 621–4.
37. Beighley PS, Brown GR, Thompson JW, Jr. DSM-III-R brief reactive psychosis among Air Force recruits. *Journal of Clinical Psychiatry* 1992; 53(8): 283–8.
38. Deakins DE, Baggett JC, Bohnker BK. Brief reactive psychosis in naval aviation. *Aviation Space and Environmental Medicine* 1991; 62(12): 1166–70.
39. Weller MP. Hysterical behaviour in patriarchal communities. Four cases, one with Ganser-like symptoms. *British Journal of Psychiatry* 1988; 152: 687–95.
40. de Kom AA, Bleeker JA. Acute reactive psychosis among immigrants in Amsterdam. *Lancet* 1991; 337(8734): 185–6.
41. Krieger MJ, Zussman M. The importance of cultural factors in a brief reactive psychosis. *Journal of Clinical Psychiatry* 1981; 42(6): 248–9.
42. Mahendran R, Aw SC. Psychiatric illness in Filipino maids admitted to Woodbridge Hospital. *Singapore Medical Journal* 1993; 34(1): 38–40.
43. Looi JC, Drew LR. Homeless, helpless and hospitalised: the travails of a Chinese refugee. *Australia and New Zealand Journal of Psychiatry* 1996; 30(5): 694–7.
44. Talmon Y, Guy N, Mayor K, Raps A, Naor S. ['Saddam syndrome:' acute psychotic reactions during the Gulf War – renewal of concept of brief reactive psychosis]. *Harefuah* 1992; 123(7–8): 237–40, 308.
45. Kapur RL, Pandurangi AK. A comparative study of reactive psychosis and acute psychosis without precipitating stress. *British Journal of Psychiatry* 1979; 135: 544–50.

46. Pandurangi AK, Kapur RL. Reactive psychosis. A prospective study. *Acta Psychiatrica Scandinavica* 1980; 61(2): 89–95.
47. Chavan BS, Kulhara P. A clinical study of reactive psychosis. *Acta Psychiatrica Scandinavica* 1988; 78(6): 712–715.
48. Chavan BS, Kulhara P. Outcome of reactive psychosis: a prospective study from India. *Acta Psychiatrica Scandinavica* 1988; 77(4): 477–82.
49. Guinness EA. Brief reactive psychosis and the major functional psychoses: descriptive case studies in Africa. *British Journal of Psychiatry Supplement* 1992; 16: 24–41.
50. Guinness EA. Relationship between the neuroses and brief reactive psychosis: descriptive case studies in Africa. *British Journal of Psychiatry Supplement* 1992; 16: 12–23.
51. Aghanwa HS, Morakinyo O, Aina OF. Consultation-liaison psychiatry in a general hospital setting in west Africa. *East Africa Medical Journal* 1996; 73(2): 133–6.
52. Collins PY, Varma VK, Wig NN, Mojtabai R, Day R, Susser E. Fever and acute brief psychosis in urban and rural settings in north India. *British Journal of Psychiatry* 1999; 174: 520–4.
53. Collins PY, Wig NN, Day R, Varma VK, Malhotra S, Misra AK, et al. Psychosocial and biological aspects of acute brief psychoses in three developing country sites. *Psychiatric Quarterly* 1996; 67(3): 177–93.
54. Bebbington P, Wilkins S, Jones P, Foerster A, Murray R, Toone B. Lewis S Life events and psychosis. Initial results from the Camberwell Collaborative Psychosis Study. *British Journal of Psychiatry* 1993; 162: 72–9.
55. Hollender MH, Hirsch SJ. Hysterical psychosis. *American Journal of Psychiatry* 1964; 120: 1066–74.
56. Langness LL. Hysterical psychosis: the cross-cultural evidence. *American Journal of Psychiatry* 1967; 124(2): 143–52.
57. Gift TE, Strauss JS, Young Y. Hysterical psychosis: an empirical approach. *American Journal of Psychiatry* 1985; 142(3): 345–7.
58. Chinchilla A, López-Ibor JJ, Cebollada A, Carrasco JL, Vega M, Jordá L, et al. [Hysterical psychosis: clinical aspects and disease course]. *Actas luso-españolas de neurología, psiquiatría y ciencias afines* 1989; 17(4): 231–6.
59. Kuruvilla K, Sitalakshmi N. Hysterical psychosis. *Indian Journal of Psychiatry* 1982; 24: 352–9.
60. Yap P. *Comparative Psychiatry*. Toronto: University of Toronto Press; 1974.
61. Haenel T. [Psychogenic psychoses]. *Schweizer Archiv für Neurologie, Neurochirurgie und Psychiatrie = Archives suisses de neurologie, neurochirurgie et de psychiatrie* 1984 ; 135(2): 299–313.
62. Spiegel D, Fink R. Hysterical psychosis and hypnotizability. *American Journal of Psychiatry* 1979; 136(6): 777–81.
63. Steingard S, Frankel FH. Dissociation and psychotic symptoms. *American Journal of Psychiatry* 1985; 142(8): 953–5.
64. Birmes P, Arrieu A, Warner B, Payen A, Moron P, Schmitt L. [Acute peritraumatic dissociative experiences: assessment and course]. *Encephale* 1999; 25(3): 18–21.
65. Magnan V. *Leçons Cliniques Sur Les Maladies Mentales*. Paris: Batielle; 1893.
66. Sutter J, Blumen G, Guin Pea. Psychoses delirantes aigues. *Encycl Med Chir Psychiatrie*, Paris 1974 ; 4(37230): A10.

67. Johnson-Sabine EC, Mann AH, Jacoby RJ, Wood KH, Peron-Magnan P, Olie JP, et al. Bouffee delirante: an examination of its current status. *Psychological Medicine* 1983; 13(4): 771–8.
68. Metzger JWH. 1991. (Cited from Garrebe J & Cousin F-R. Acute and Transient Psychotic Disorders p 649. In MG Gelder, JJ Lopez-Ibor, Nancy Andreasen. *Oxford Textbook of Psychiatry*, Oxford University Press, 2000)
69. Ferrey G, Zebdi S. [The development and prognosis of acute psychotic disorders (polymorphic delirium flushes)]. *Encephale* 1999; 25(3): 26–32.
70. Priest RG, Laffont I. [The British and French systems of classification and psychiatric disorders]. *Annals of Medical Psychology (Paris)* 1992; 150(4–5): 313–317.
71. Fukuda T. Cycloid psychoses as atypical psychoses: 'concordance' and 'discordance'. *Psychopathology* 1990; 23(4–6): 253–8.
72. Hatotani N. The concept of 'atypical psychoses': special reference to its development in Japan. *Psychiatry and Clinical Neuroscience* 1996; 50(1): 1–10.
73. Cooper JE, Jablensky A, Sartorius N. WHO Collaborative studies on acute psychoses using the SCAAPS schedule. In: Steffanis CR, Soldatos AD, editors. *Psychiatry: a world perspective*. Amsterdam: Elsevier Science Publishers; 1990, p. 185–192.
74. Okasha A. Problems of schizo-affective disorders. *Psychiatrica Clinica (Basel)* 1983; 16(2–4): 149–55.
75. Okasha A, el Dawla AS, Khalil AH, Saad A. Presentation of acute psychosis in an Egyptian sample: a transcultural comparison. *Comprehensive Psychiatry* 1993; 34(1): 4–9.
76. Susser E, Varma VK, Malhotra S, Conover S, Amador XF. Delineation of acute and transient psychotic disorders in a developing country setting. *British Journal of Psychiatry* 1995; 167(2): 216–19.
77. Susser E, Varma VK, Mattoo SK, Finnerty M, Mojtabai R, Tripathi BM, et al. Long-term course of acute brief psychosis in a developing country setting. *British Journal of Psychiatry* 1998; 173: 226–30.
78. Jablensky A, Sartorius N, Ernberg G, Anker M, Korten A, Cooper JE, et al. Schizophrenia: manifestations, incidence and course in different cultures. A World Health Organization ten-country study. *Psychological Medicine Monograph* Supplement 1992; 20: 1–97.
79. Sartorius N, Jablensky A, Shapiro R. Cross-cultural differences in the short-term prognosis of schizophrenic psychoses. *Schizophrenia Bulletin* 1978; 4(1): 102–13.
80. Varma VK, Brown AS, Wig NN, Tripathi BM, Misra AK, Khare CB, et al. Effects of level of socio-economic development on course of non-affective psychosis. *British Journal of Psychiatry* 1997; 171: 256–9.
81. Allodi F. Acute paranoid reaction (bouffee delirante) in Canada. *Canadian Journal of Psychiatry* 1982; 27(5): 366–73.
82. Pichot P. The concept of 'bouffee delirante' with special reference to the Scandinavian concept of reactive psychosis. *Psychopathology* 1986; 19(1–2): 35–43.
83. Leonhard K. Prognosis of paranoid states in relation to the clinical features. *Acta Psychiatrica Scandinavica* 1975; 51(2): 134–51.
84. Modestin J, Bachmann KM. Is the diagnosis of hysterical psychosis justified? Clinical study of hysterical psychosis, reactive/psychogenic psychosis, and schizophrenia. *Comprehensive Psychiatry* 1992; 33(1): 17–24.

85. Vaillant GE. The prediction of recovery in schizophrenia. *Journal of Nervous and Mental Disorder* 1962; 135: 534–43.

86. Vaillant GE. A 10-year followup of remitting schizophrenics. *Schizophrenia Bulletin* 1978; 4(1): 78–85.

87. Vaillant GE. An historical review of the remitting schizophrenias. *Journal of Nervous and Mental Disorder* 1964; 138: 48–56.

88. Vaillant GE. The natural history of the remitting schizophrenias. *American Journal of Psychiatry* 1963; 120: 367–76.

89. Westermeyer JF, Harrow M. Prognosis and outcome using broad (DSM-II) and narrow (DSM-III) concepts of schizophrenia. *Schizophrenia Bulletin* 1984; 10(4): 624–37.

90. Singh SP, Cooper JE, Fisher HL et al. Determining the chronology and components of psychosis onset: the Nottingham Onset Schedule (NOS). *Schizophrenia Research* 2005; 80: 117–30.

91. Bergem AL, Dahl AA, Guldberg C, Hansen H. Langfeldt's schizophreniform psychoses fifty years later. *British Journal of Psychiatry* 1990; 157: 351–4.

92. Strakowski SM. Diagnostic validity of schizophreniform disorder. *American Journal of Psychiatry* 1994; 151(6): 815–24.

93. Langfeldt G. Definition of 'schizophreniform psychoses'. *American Journal of Psychiatry* 1982; 139(5): 703.

94. Beiser M, Erickson D, Fleming JA, Iacono WG. Establishing the onset of psychotic illness. *American Journal of Psychiatry* 1993; 150(9): 1349–54.

95. Zhang-Wong J, Beiser M, Bean G, Iacono WG. Five-year course of schizophreniform disorder. *Psychiatry Research* 1995; 59(1–2): 109–17.

96. Guldberg CA, Dahl AA, Hansen H, Bergem AL. Were Langfeldt's schizophreniform psychoses really affective? *Psychopathology* 1991; 24(5): 270–6.

97. Guldberg CA, Dahl AA, Hansen H, Bergem M. Predictive value of the four good prognostic features in DSM-III-R schizophreniform disorder. *Acta Psychiatrica Scandinavica* 1990; 82(1): 23–5.

98. Huber G, Gross G, Schuttler R, Linz M.Longitudinal studies of schizophrenic patients. *Schizophrenia Bulletin* 1980; 6(4): 592–605.

99. Armbruster B, Gross G, Huber G. Long-term prognosis and course of schizo-affective, schizophreniform, and cycloid psychoses. *Psychiatrica Clinica (Basel)* 1983; 16(2–4): 156–68.

100. Amin S, Singh SP, Brewin J, Jones PB, Medley I, Harrison G. Diagnostic stability of first-episode psychosis. Comparison of ICD-10 and DSM-III-R systems. *British Journal of Psychiatry* 1999; 175: 537–43.

101. Johnstone EC, Connelly J, Frith CD, Lambert MT, Owens DG.The nature of 'transient' and 'partial' psychoses: findings from the Northwick Park 'Functional' Psychosis Study. *Psychological Medicine* 1996; 26(2): 361–9.

102. Keith S J, Matthews S M (1991) The diagnosis of schizophrenia: a review of onset and duration issues. *Schizophr Bull,* 17: 51-67

103. McGalshan (1988) A selective review of recent North American long-term followup studies of schizophrenia. *Schizophr Bull* 14: 515-42

104. Susser E, Finnerty MT, Sohler N. Acute psychoses: a proposed diagnosis for ICD-11 and DSM-V. *Psychiatric Quarterly* 1996; 67(3): 165–76.

105. Mojtabai R, Susser ES, Bromet EJ. Clinical characteristics, 4-year course, and DSM-IV classification of patients with nonaffective acute remitting psychosis. *American Journal of Psychiatry* 2003; 160(12): 2108–115.

106. Mojtabai R, Varma VK, Susser E. Duration of remitting psychoses with acute onset. Implications for ICD-10. *British Journal of Psychiatry* 2000; 176: 576–80.

107. Andreasen NC, Carpenter WT, Jr., Kane JM, Lasser RA, Marder SR, Weinberger DR. Remission in schizophrenia: proposed criteria and rationale for consensus. *American Journal of Psychiatry* 2005; 162(3): 441–9.

108. Marneros A, Pillmann F, Haring A, Balzuweit S, Bloink R. What is schizophrenic in acute and transient psychotic disorder? *Schizophrenia Bulletin* 2003; 29(2): 311–23.

109. Marneros A, Pillmann F, Haring A, Balzuweit S, Bloink R. Features of acute and transient psychotic disorders. *European Archives of Psychiatry and Clinical Neuroscience* 2003; 253(4): 167–74.

110. Jorgensen P, Bennedsen B, Christensen J, Hyllested A. Acute and transient psychotic disorder: a 1-year follow-up study. *Acta Psychiatrica Scandinavica* 1997; 96(2): 150–4.

111. Susser E, Fennig S, Jandorf L, Amador X, Bromet E. Epidemiology, diagnosis, and course of brief psychoses. *American Journal of Psychiatry* 1995; 152(12): 1743–8.

112. Modestin J, Sonderegger P, Erni T. Follow-up study of hysterical psychosis, reactive/psychogenic psychosis, and schizophrenia. *Comprehensive Psychiatry* 2001; 42(1): 51–6.

113. Pitta JC, Blay SL. Psychogenic (reactive) and hysterical psychoses: a cross-system reliability study. *Acta Psychiatrica Scandinavica* 1997; 95(2): 112–118.

114. McGorry PD, Singh BS, Connell S, McKenzie D, Van Riel RJ, Copolov DL. Diagnostic concordance in functional psychosis revisited: a study of inter-relationships between alternative concepts of psychotic disorder. *Psychological Medicine* 1992; 22(2): 367–78.

115. Hansen H, Dahl AA, Bertelsen A, Birket-Smith M, von Knorring L, Ottosson JO, et al. The Nordic concept of reactive psychosis--a multicenter reliability study. *Acta Psychiatrica Scandinavica* 1992; 86(1): 55–9.

116. Pichot PJ. DSM-III and its reception: a European view. *American Journal of Psychiatry* 1997; 154(6 Suppl): 47–54.

117. McGorry PD, Mihalopoulos C, Henry L, Dakis J, Jackson HJ, Flaum M, et al. Spurious precision: procedural validity of diagnostic assessment in psychotic disorders. *American Journal of Psychiatry* 1995; 152(2): 220–3.

118. Jablensky A. Classification of nonschizophrenic psychotic disorders: a historical perspective. *Current Psychiatry Report* 2001; 3(4): 326–31.

119. Tsuang MT, Stone WS. Faraone SV. Toward reformulating the diagnosis of schizophrenia. *American Journal of Psychiatry* 2000; 157(7): 1041–50.

120. Hiller W, Dichtl G, Hecht H, Hundt W, von Zerssen D. Testing the comparability of psychiatric diagnoses in ICD-10 and DSM-III-R. *Psychopathology* 1994; 27(1–2): 19–28.

121. Kendell RE, Brockington IF, Leff JP. Prognostic implications of six alternative definitions of schizophrenia. *Archives of General Psychiatry* 1979; 36(1): 25–31.

122. McGuffin P et al. Twin concordance for operationally defined schizophrenia. Confirmation of familiality and heritability. *Archives of General Psychiatry* 1984; 41(6): 541–5.

123. Taylor MA. Are schizophrenia and affective disorder related? A selective literature review. *American Journal of Psychiatry* 1992; 149(1): 22–32.
124. Taylor MA, Amir N. Are schizophrenia and affective disorder related? The problem of schizoaffective disorder and the discrimination of the psychoses by signs and symptoms. *Comprehensive Psychiatry* 1994; 35(6): 420–9.
125. Taylor MA, Berenbaum SA, Jampala VC, Cloninger CR. Are schizophrenia and affective disorder related? preliminary data from a family study. *American Journal of Psychiatry* 1993; 150(2): 278–85.
126. Faraone SV, Blehar M, Pepple J, Moldin SO, Norton J, Nurnberger JI, et al. Diagnostic accuracy and confusability analyses: an application to the Diagnostic Interview for Genetic Studies. *Psychological Medicine* 1996; 26(2): 401–410.
127. Munro A. Neither lions nor tigers: disorders which lie between schizophrenia and affective disorder. *Canadian Journal of Psychiatry* 1987; 32(4): 296–7.
128. Castle DJ, Sham PC, Wessely S, Murray RM. The subtyping of schizophrenia in men and women: a latent class analysis. *Psychological Medicine* 1994; 24(1): 41–51.
129. Kendler KS, Walsh D. The structure of psychosis: syndromes and dimensions. *Archives of General Psychiatry* 1998; 55(6): 508–509.
130. Peralta V, Cuesta MJ. How many and which are the psychopathological dimensions in schizophrenia? Issues influencing their ascertainment. *Schizophrenia Research* 2001; 49(3): 269–85.
131. van Os J, Verdoux H, Maurice-Tison S, Gay B, Liraud F, Salamon R, et al. Self-reported psychosis-like symptoms and the continuum of psychosis. *Social Psychiatry and Psychiatric Epidemiology* 1999 ; 34(9): 459–63.
132. Kitamura T, Okazaki Y, Fujinawa A, Yoshino M, Kasahara Y. Symptoms of psychoses. A factor-analytic study. *British Journal of Psychiatry* 1995; 166(2): 236–40.
133. van Os J, Fahy TA, Jones P, Harvey I, Sham P, Lewis S, et al. Psychopathological syndromes in the functional psychoses: associations with course and outcome. *Psychological Medicine* 1996; 26(1): 161–76.
134. Castle DJ, Murray RM. The neurodevelopmental basis of sex differences in schizophrenia. *Psychological Medicine* 1991; 21(3): 565–75.
135. Fisch RZ. Psychosis precipitated by marriage: a culture-bound syndrome? *British Journal of Medical Psychology* 1992; 65(Pt 4): 385–91.
136. Mezzisch JE, Lin KM. Acute and transient psychotic disorders and culture-bound syndromes. In: Kaplan HS, Kaplan B, editors. *Comprehensive Textbook of Psychiatry*. Baltimore: Williams and Wilkins; 1995, p. 1049–57.
137. Kirmayer LJ, Groleau D. Affective disorders in cultural context. *Psychiatric Clinics of North America* 2001; 24(3): 465–78, vii.
138. Kirmayer LJ, Young A, Hayton BC. The cultural context of anxiety disorders. *Psychiatric Clinics of North America* 1995; 18(3): 503–21.

Part II

Interface of Medicine and Psychiatry

6
Symptoms Unexplained by Disease

Alan Carson and Jon Stone

Symptoms such as pain, weakness, fatigue and sensory disturbance often lack a disease explanation. Such symptoms can be a major problem for both doctor and patient, often challenging the way in which we conceptualise and practise medicine. Symptoms are the patient's subjective experience of what is occurring in their body. By contrast, doctors are trained to find diseases such as multiple sclerosis that offer an explanation for these symptoms. When there is no disease present it becomes tempting to suggest that the symptom is not real or psychogenic. However, symptoms appear for multiple reasons, including physiological factors, psychological factors, behavioural response and cultural and social factors. For some patients disease pathology is a major factor in causing symptoms but in others it appears to be minor or absent entirely. A patient does not have to have a disease in order to have genuine symptoms.

In this article we borrow explicitly from a previous review on the topic,[1,2] but have oriented this article more to psychiatric rather than neurological practice.

Terminology

The confusion surrounding this area is reflected in the myriad of descriptive terms for symptoms that are unexplained by disease. This is in part a reflection of the diverse number of concepts that are being used to understand them. There are descriptive labels such as chronic fatigue or low back pain, sometimes elevated to symptom syndromes such as chronic fatigue syndrome or irritable bowel syndrome. Negative diagnoses describe what the diagnosis is *not* rather than what it is, for instance, non-epileptic attack, non-organic or medically unexplained symptoms. Some diagnoses suggest an as yet non-established disease cause, for example, reflex sympathetic dystrophy. Others suggest a purely psychological cause such as psychogenic dystonia.

There are operationalised psychiatric diagnoses such as conversion disorder (*Diagnostic and Statistical Manual of Mental Disorders* [4th edition; DSM-IV]), and dissociative disorder (*International Classification of Diseases* [10th edition; ICD-10]) but these suffer from criteria that are very hard to use in practice. For example, it is difficult to prove the absence of wilful simulation and the relevance of psychological factors (in the case of conversion disorder). Somatisation disorder is a diagnosis that is easier to apply in practice and of more clinical use, describing as it does a pattern starting before the age of 30 years with repeated presentations with different symptoms unexplained by disease (one neurological, four pain, two gastrointestinal and one sexual). A ragbag of other labels including hysteria, and functional symptoms complete the range of terms available. We discuss how to handle the issue of terminology with the patient later in this chapter.

What most of these terms have in common is the concept that the patient's presentation is genuine and that they are not trying to deceive their doctor. As such, this group of disorders need to be distinguished from factitious disorders and malingering. Factitious disorder refers to presentations in which the patient has deliberately falsified clinical symptoms, and sometimes signs, in order to deceive their doctor. This is done consciously and with the full knowledge that deception is taking place. The motive for this behaviour is the desire for medical attention. This is generally contrasted with malingering, which involves the same behaviour but where the motive is financial gain. Perhaps not surprisingly, there is a strong association between factitious disorder and severe personality disorder.

Epidemiology

A major constraint to studying the epidemiology of unexplained symptoms is deciding what one is actually going to examine. Thus, a study that looks at the prevalence of any symptom of fatigue in the population will find different results to a study looking at disabling fatigue (however transient), to a study looking at persistent and disabling fatigue, i.e. a chronic fatigue syndrome, to a study looking at somatoform disorders, etc. Nonetheless, however one chooses to look at and define the problem, what is clear is that symptoms unexplained by disease are common and make up a large part of medical practice.

To some extent, physical symptoms such as mild tiredness, occasional headache and transient back pain are so common that they can be regarded as normal. If one limits the sample using disability criteria to those patients where the complaint is substantial, one still finds that between 10 and 20% of the population complain of fatigue and neck pain and 5–10% complain of headache.

Using investigation to refine studies of such patients may bring about its own problems. Take the example of spinal imaging for back pain. Some of the 'abnormalities' that may be reported are so common in people with *no* back pain that they are clinically impossible to interpret. In studies of asymptomatic patients, disk herniation occurs in over 20% of subjects and disc bulging in over 50%. Over the age of 60 years, over 90% of people have degenerative changes on a spinal magnetic resonance imaging (MRI).[3]

An alternative approach is to use psychiatrically derived definitions from the DSM or ICD. The epidemiological catchment area study found the presence of undifferentiated somatoform disorder (two or more significant functional symptoms or syndromes) to be around 4% and of somatisation disorder to be around 0.1%.[4]

Given that a major feature of unexplained symptoms is help-seeking behaviour, clearly the setting in which the sample is derived will influence the prevalence rate. The World Health Organization's (WHO's) international study conducted in general practice settings in 15 separate countries found that undifferentiated somatoform disorder had a prevalence of around 20% and somatisation disorder a prevalence of around 3%.[5] What was of particular interest was that the rates were similar in most countries worldwide.

Kroenke and colleagues took a different approach to the problem and studied the rates of individual symptoms reported in a primary care setting. They then demonstrated that only a low proportion of each individual symptom had a defined pathological explanation (Figure 6.1).[6]

In a secondary care setting, numerous studies have consistently shown that around one-third of new presentations to doctors are for symptoms that are unexplained by disease. The nature of the presentations will vary depending upon the outpatient clinics studied (Table 6.1).

It has been frequently claimed that the nature of the presentation of unexplained symptoms has changed substantially over time, with a particular emphasis placed on the diminished prevalence of conversion disorders. The evidence to support these claims is in fact weak. Charcot in 1890 found that 8% of his outpatients had hysteria. Figures for the frequency of conversion symptoms in modern-day neurological

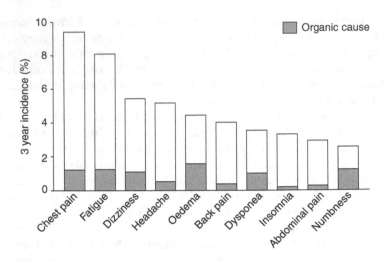

Figure 6.1   The proportion of symptoms in primary care explained by disease

Source: Reproduced with permission from Kroenke K, Mangelsdorff AD. Common symptoms in ambulatory care: incidence, evaluation, therapy, and outcome. *American Journal of Medicine* 1989; 86(3): 262–6.[6]

Table 6.1   Symptoms and syndromes unexplained by disease in different medical specialties

Specialty	Symptom/syndrome
Neurology	Functional weakness, non-epileptic attacks, hemisensory symptoms
Gastroenterology	Irritable bowel syndrome, non-ulcer dyspepsia, chronic abdominal pain
Gynaecology	Chronic pelvic pain, premenstrual syndrome
Ear nose and throat	Functional dysphonia, globus pharynges
Cardiology	Atypical chest pain, unexplained palpitations
Rheumatology	Fibromyalgia
Infectious diseases	(Post-viral) chronic fatigue syndrome
Immunology/allergy	Multiple chemical sensitivity syndrome

outpatients are similar.[7] Incidence figures for functional paralysis of approximately 5 per 100,000 have been described, i.e. similar to multiple sclerosis.[8] Thus, the claims that such disorders are rare and largely historical conditions do not appear to be supported. Similarly, non-epileptic attacks, still account for about 10–20% of patients referred to specialist epilepsy clinics with intractable seizures and up to 50% of patients admitted to hospital in apparent status epilepticus.[9]

A major concern in epidemiological investigation has been the issue of misdiagnosis. In a very influential paper in the 1960s, Eliot Slater claimed that somewhere between one-third and two-thirds of patients diagnosed with what he described as hysteria turned out to have organic disease explanations for their symptoms if followed up. A recent systematic review demonstrated a consistently described misdiagnosis rate of around 4–5% since 1970.[10] This rate of 'misdiagnosis' is no different from any other neurological or psychiatric disorder and also predates the computed tomography (CT) scan, emphasising that diagnosis remains dependent upon history and examination (Figure 6.2).

Prognosis

There are only a limited number of prognostic studies looking at patient outcome and most are small. Nonetheless, despite marked heterogeneity in the samples, the majority of studies, seem to suggest that around half of patients will go into remission in the first year after diagnosis. Factors

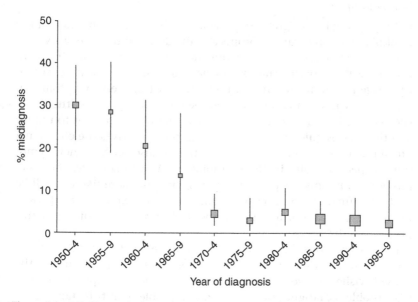

Figure 6.2 Misdiagnosis is no more common than for other neurological and psychiatric disorders (around 5% since 1970) – systematic review of 27 studies and 1466 patients

Source: Reproduced with permission from Stone J, Smyth R, Carson A et al. Systematic review of misdiagnosis of conversion symptoms and 'hysteria'. *BMJ* 2005; 331(7523): 989.[10]

that may be associated with better outcome are changes in life circumstances during the follow-up period (e.g. a marriage or divorce), illness beliefs that improvement is likely, lack of illness-dependent financial benefits and better premorbid function.

For patients who do not improve early on, the evidence from very long term follow-up studies suggests that the majority of patients, perhaps around 50–75% tend to stay symptomatic on a long-term basis.[11]

Clinical assessment of the patient with symptoms unexplained by disease

We will describe our practical approach to history taking and examination, paying particular attention to the use of positive physical signs in diagnosis, not just the absence of disease. We will use the examples of paralysis, non-epileptic attacks and back pain. More detailed guidance can be found elsewhere.[1]

Taking the history

List the symptoms

History taking in this group of patients can be daunting because of the multiplicity of physical symptoms and the duration of the history

We suggest beginning the history taking by making a long list of all the physical symptoms the patient has suffered. It is not necessary at this stage to interrogate the features and onset of every symptom but, rather, a few lines should be left between each symptom on the list so they can be returned to as required. This allows the patient to unburden themselves quickly of all their symptoms and gives the clinician a broad picture early on in the consultation. It also prevents new symptoms 'appearing' later in the consultation. As a broad rule, the more physical symptoms the patient presents with the more likely it will be that the primary presenting symptom will not be explained by disease. Encourage the patient to tell you about all possible symptoms at this point, even dizziness!

Even if the consultation is explicitly a psychiatric one, resist the temptation to ask about emotional symptoms at this point, unless the patient wishes to. Do, however, ask about somatic symptoms such as sleep problems, fatigue and concentration problems at this stage

Ask about disability

Ask the patient to describe 'what is a typical day like?'. Follow up with questions such as 'how much of the day do you spend in bed?' and 'how often do you leave the house?'. These are generally more useful than traditional disability questions about dressing and walking distance. Ask yourself why the patient is disabled. For example, a mild hemiparesis may not impair gait but may cause a fear of falling, which is why they do not go outside.

Ask about dissociation

Dissociative symptoms include depersonalisation (feeling detached from oneself) and derealisation (feeling that the world is no longer real). These occur in a range of disorders such as epilepsy, migraine and, less commonly, in healthy individuals. They also occur quite commonly in patients with unexplained neurological symptoms, particularly those who have experienced paralysis and non-epileptic attacks. Patients may say, 'I felt as if I was there, but not there, as if I was outside of myself'; 'I was spaced out, in a place of my own'; 'things around me didn't feel real, it was like I was watching everything on television'; 'my body didn't feel like my own'; 'I couldn't see but I could hear everyone. I just couldn't reply'. These symptoms often occur in an anxiety or panic attack, although patients often have not made this connection.

Patients frequently find it difficult to describe dissociation and may just say they feel dizzy, or indeed be frightened of raising the topic at all as they believe the symptom may indicated 'madness'. They are often relieved to discover that the symptoms are common and nothing to do with going mad. The experience of dissociation can be used to explain to patients the link between their experiences and the development of unusual symptoms such as a limb no longer feeling as if it is part of them.

What happened with previous doctors?

Ask the patient to tell you about doctors whom they saw previously. They may complain bitterly about Doctor X who 'didn't listen to them' or who told them it was 'nothing serious'. You should not get involved in commenting upon Doctor X's practice but you should listen closely to the content. First, it may serve to warn about symptom explanations and treatments that are likely to be rejected or perceived as offensive. Second, by letting the patient talk openly about the previous disappointing medical encounters, you are showing them your interest in their suffering and attempting to understand their frustration. This point was best made by Nortin Hadler with the comment 'if you have to prove you are ill you cannot get well'.[12]

Ask about their illness beliefs

What does the patient think is causing their symptoms? Do they think they are reversible or irreversible? What do they think should be done about them? Are they really worried about the possibility of serious disease? This last question is especially useful in deciding to what extent the patient has health anxiety (also known as hypochondriasis). The severity of health anxiety ranges hugely in these patients. The approach to treatment will vary quite a lot depending on this. For example, patients with severe health anxiety seek reassurance, which is only short lived and their reassurance seeking will need to be addressed openly. Patients with no anxiety do not need this approach

There is an increasing body of evidence that patients' illness cognitions do influence outcome and are essential for guiding the initial stages of any treatment based on cognitive-behavioural principles

Past medical history

The more functional symptoms or syndromes (Table 6.1) a patient has had in the past, the more likely it is that their current symptoms are also functional. There may also be a history of medical attempts to treat these symptoms with surgical operations (for example hysterectomy at a young age, appendicectomy with a normal specimen, laparoscopy to investigate abdominal pain). Patients may not always remember or want to tell you about previous symptoms unexplained by disease (and especially psychiatric history), out of concern that this will make their current symptoms less credible. For this reason, it is particularly helpful to review old case notes in complex presentations. If the patient has already had a disease diagnosis, always consider whether the evidence recorded in the case notes justifies it.

Social history

Work, money, the law and marriage, an unpleasant job, being in a state benefit trap and involvement in a legal case can all be relevant obstacles to recovery. This should not be instantly assumed as being the cause of the symptoms but it is important to understand in terms of assessing outcome. Do not be put off if you cannot find a relevant life event in patients with new-onset symptoms. There may not be one, in the same way that a patient with new-onset panic disorder may not have a relevant life event either.

Emotional symptoms

Numerous studies have demonstrated that depression, anxiety and panic disorder are much more common in patients with symptoms unexplained by disease than those patients with disease. In general, studies have found that the more physical symptoms the patient has, the more emotional symptoms they will have too. However, asking about psychological symptoms can be a minefield and patients frequently become defensive.

You will hopefully have some clues already after asking about somatic symptoms such as fatigue, poor concentration and poor sleep. When asking about emotional symptoms, it may help to frame the question in terms of the symptoms the patient presented with and try to avoid psychiatric terms such as depression, anxiety and panic. For example, instead of asking 'have you been feeling depressed?', try 'do your symptoms ever make you feel down or frustrated?'. Instead of 'do you enjoy things any more?', try 'how much of the time do your symptoms stop you enjoying things?'. When the patient replies that they can't enjoy things because they can't walk, ask them how often they can enjoy the things they can do, such as watching television.

If you suspect your patient has been having panic attacks or is agoraphobic, ask 'do you have attacks where you have lots of symptoms all at once, when does this happen, is it when you are outside or in certain situations?'. It is important to remember that many patients, not just those with functional symptoms, regard anything psychological as a sign of mental weakness, madness or an accusation of making up symptoms. Therefore it cannot be emphasised enough how important it is to be careful about such questions of psychological symptoms. We have found that once the patient trusts that you are not going to use emotional symptoms 'against' them, they often tell you important things they might not otherwise have done.

Personal history

Childhood abuse and neglect is another important factor that makes people more prone to functional symptoms. However, it is difficult to know, particularly at a first consultation, to what extent one should enquire about these symptoms. Use your clinical judgement in taking cues from the patient and whether they are dropping 'hints' that you should ask. Otherwise, we would certainly recommend being cautious about asking about abuse, at least until subsequent consultations, even if the history is strongly suggestive. The current evidence, particularly from primary care, does not support the idea that exploring these things superficially will necessarily improve outcome.[13]

The physical examination

The diagnosis of unexplained symptoms, with respect to neurological symptoms anyway, depends upon demonstrating both positive signs of conversion symptoms and the absence of signs of disease. The physical diagnosis of these conditions is difficult and should be made by the appropriate specialist (e.g. neurologist, gastroenterologist). However, even if you are seeing the patient as a psychiatrist, we suggest that these positive signs are useful to learn and show to patients and should be part of a routine assessment.

Most of these positive signs relate to inconsistency, either internal (for example Hoover's sign reveals discrepancies in leg power), or external (for example a tubular field defect that is inconsistent with the laws of optics). These signs do not tell you whether the symptoms are consciously or unconsciously produced. The presence of a positive sign also does not exclude the possibility that the patient also has disease – they may have both. Finally, all physical signs have limited sensitivity, specificity and inter-rater reliability.

General signs

Demonstrative pain behaviour at the time of history such as rubbing oneself continually, grimacing, and groaning raises the likelihood that symptoms are unexplained but are dangerous to use in isolation. 'La belle indifference', an apparent lack of concern about the nature, implications of symptoms and disability, has little discriminatory value.[14] In our own experience, patients who are said to have la belle indifference are usually making an effort to appear cheerful in a conscious attempt not to be labelled as depressed, or have subsequently been shown to have factitious disorders.

Weakness

General evidence of inconsistency may be found, for example a marked difference in gait when a patient leaves the consulting room compared to when they came in. They may use a limb very differently when removing clothes or getting something from their bag.

Hoover's sign is a useful test for 'functional' paralysis, with a small amount of data to support its use. The test relies on the principle that we extend our hip when flexing our contralateral hip against resistance. Patients with functional paralysis often have weakness of hip extension but this returns to normal when testing contralateral hip flexion against resistance. This is a sign you can try out on yourself in the seated position (Figure 6.3). Pain and cortical neglect could cause a positive Hoover sign, and the test may be mildly positive in normal individuals because of a splinting effect.

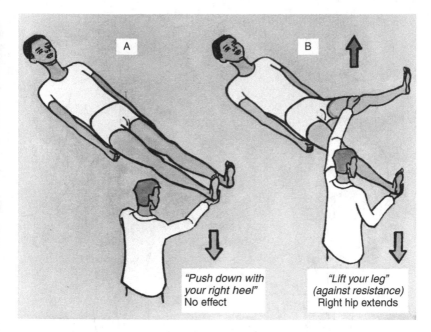

Figure 6.3   Hoover's sign to test for functional weakness

Source: Reproduced with permission from Stone J, Carson A, Sharpe M. Functional symptoms and signs in neurology: assessment and diagnosis. *Journal of Neurology Neurosurgery and Psychiatry* 2005; 76(Suppl 1): i–i12. [1]

Another positive sign is collapsing weakness, in which a limb collapses with light touch, often associated with intermittent power. Normal power may be observed transiently with encouragement or for short periods of time. A patient's inability to understand instructions for an examination, general malaise, or a misguided eagerness to convince the doctor may cause false results here, and this is probably not as useful as Hoover's sign. Further signs are described elsewhere.[15]

Sensory disturbance

Patients may describe sensory loss that ends with the leg ends or ends where the arm ends.

More commonly patients describe feeling 'cut in half' with one side of their body just feeling different to the other side (Figure 6.4).

Tests are described for sensory symptoms such as 'midline splitting', in which the finding of exact splitting of sensation in the midline is

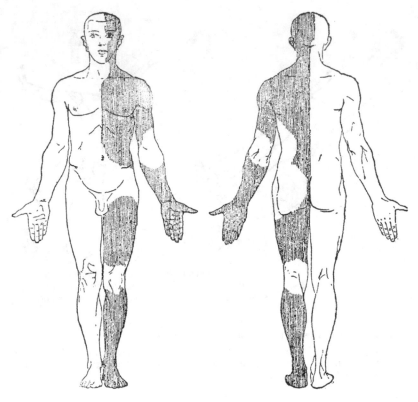

Figure 6.4 Hemisensory disturbance

Source: Reproduced with permission from Charcot JM. *Clinical Lectures on Diseases of the Nervous System* (Volume 3). London: New Sydenham Society; 1889.[16]

said to be a positive sign inconsistent with disease (as the branches of intercostal nerves overlap the midline). Similarly, patients might not expect a difference in sensation of a tuning fork placed over the left compared to the right side of the sternum or frontal bone, as the bone is a single unit and should vibrate as one. However, studies have tended to show these signs, like all sensory tests in neurology, are unreliable. Sensory signs are therefore worth noting but should not be relied upon to make a diagnosis.

Non-epileptic attacks

There are a large number of clinical features which, in combination, can be used to distinguish non-epileptic attacks from epilepsy

(Table 6.2).[9] In practice however, this distinction may be very difficult, relying as it often does on unreliable witness histories. Many types of epileptic attack, especially frontal lobe seizures, may look 'psychogenic'. The diagnosis should only be made by someone with a lot of experience of diagnosing epilepsy. Videotelemetry allows for a more confident diagnosis (although some frontal lobe seizures may be silent on the electroencephalogram [EEG]) and is useful for creating clinical confidence and to feed back to the patient and their families. Serum prolactin is more often elevated after a generalised seizure than other kinds of attack, but its sensitivity and specificity in the context of all attack disorders means that it more often confuses the clinical diagnosis than helps it. See Chapter 7 for more details on this topic.

Table 6.2 Attack features that can help to distinguish non-epileptic attacks from epileptic seizures

Observation	Non-epileptic seizures	Epileptic seizures
Situational onset	Occasional	Rare
Gradual onset	Common	Rare
Precipitated by stimuli (noise, light)	Occasional	Rare
Undulating motor activity	Common	Very rare
Asynchronous limb movements	Common	Rare
Purposeful movements	Occasional	Very rare
Rhythmic pelvic movements	Occasional	Rare
Opisthotonus, 'arc de cercle'	Occasional	Very rare
Side-to-side head shaking	Common	Rare
Tongue biting (bitemark seen)	Rare	Common
Grunting/snoring sounds	Rare	Common
Prolonged ictal atonia	Occasional	Very rare
Ictal crying	Occasional	Very rare
Closed mouth in 'tonic phase'	Occasional	Very rare
Vocalisation during 'tonic–clonic' phase	Occasional	Very rare
Closed eyelids	Very common	Rare
Convulsion >2 minutes	Common	Very rare
Resistance to eyelid opening	Common	Very rare
Pupillary light reflex	Usually retained	Commonly absent
Reactivity during 'unconsciousness'	Occasional	Very rare
Lack of cyanosis	Common	Rare
Rapid postictal reorientation	Common	Rare

Source: Reproduced with permission from Reuber M, Elger CE. Psychogenic nonepileptic seizures: review and update. *Epilepsy and Behaviour* 2003; 4(3): 205–169.

Functional movement disorders and gait disturbance

Tremor,[17] fixed postures (dystonia)[18] and exaggerated startle responses (myoclonus) are all described as forms of functional/psychogenic movement disorder.[15] Their diagnosis is especially difficult because of the often strange and inconsistent presentation of organic movement disorders such as dystonia. Typical presentations include:

   a tremor of highly variable amplitude and frequency that disappears with (or entrains to) voluntary rhythmic movements of a contralateral limb
   a clenched hand or an inverted and plantarflexed ankle, especially after injury.

Unilateral functional leg weakness tends to produce a characteristic gait in which the leg is dragged behind the body as a single unit like a log. Many other gait problems such as a 'walking on tightrope' gait and a gait with an 'uneconomic posture' are described.[19] It should be noted that functional gait problems and movement disorders are most likely, with hindsight, to turn out to be due to neurological disease.[10]

Back pain

Physical examination findings suggestive of unexplained back pain were described by Waddell and colleagues in what they called 'abnormal illness behaviour':[20]

   inconsistent performance of seated versus supine straight-leg raising test
   tenderness that was superficial or widespread, particularly to the lightest of touches, or light touch sending pain radiating up the back
   pain on simulated axial loading, i.e. putting pressure on the top of the head, or pain on simulated rotation of the pelvis and shoulder such that the spine is held on the same plane without movement
   sensory or motor findings without anatomic distribution as described above
   a general tendency to over-reaction during examination.

These signs are clinically useful but, once again, should not be relied upon too much in isolation.

Investigations

Even with positive signs that the symptoms are unexplained by disease, investigations are frequently necessary. However, unlike other fields of medicine, we often find that the desire to perform investigations is not just because of our uncertainty about the diagnosis, but sometimes because of the patient's uncertainty. We have found that some patients really do not want tests, they just want a confident opinion, but others are only interested in the opinion of a CT scanner. As a rule of thumb, we have found that if one is carrying out investigations to convince or reassure patients, this reassurance may only be temporarily effective. In patients with severe health anxiety, investigations may actually be counterproductive. When investigations are going to be conducted, they should be performed as quickly as possible and an explanation of likely outcome given to the patients in advance. This must involve a realistic assessment of the likelihood of uncovering disease balanced against the risks of laboratory and radiological abnormalities that have nothing to do with the symptoms.

Aetiology

Symptoms unexplained by disease have a long history in medicine going back to the 'wandering womb' ideas implied by the word hysteria. In the last 200 years, the debate has been largely about whether they are a product of the mind or of the brain. In the last 100 years, the psychiatric interpretation has dominated. It is increasingly clear, however, that such a debate is actually rather meaningless and that the problem can be looked at usefully from both a 'brain' perspective and a 'mind' perspective.

The aetiology of symptoms unexplained by disease can be considered in terms of biological, psychological and social factors, or it can be considered in terms of factors that predispose, precipitate and perpetuate symptoms. These factors are described in Table 6.3. Although a biopsychosocial approach is often used as a 'mantra' in considering such conditions, in our experience the biological is often dropped and the psychosocial emphasised. It is probably just as erroneous to omit consideration of biological factors as it is to ignore the psychological and social factors. Techniques such as functional imaging are helping to demonstrate the biological dimension of these symptoms (Figure 6.5).[21] These disorders are almost certainly multifactorial in their origin and

Table 6.3   A scheme for thinking about the aetiology of functional symptoms in neurology

Factors	Biological	Psychological	Social
Predisposing	• Genetic factors affecting personality • Biological vulnerabilities in the nervous system? • Disease	• Poor 'attachment' to parents and others • Personality/coping style	• Childhood neglect/abuse • Poor family functioning
Precipitating	• Abnormal physiological event or state (e.g. hyperventilation, sleep deprivation, sleep paralysis) • Physical injury/pain	• Perception of life event as negative, unexpected • Depression/anxiety • Acute dissociative episode/panic attack	• Symptom modelling (via media or personal contact) • Life events and difficulties
Perpetuating	• Plasticity in central nervous system (CNS) motor and sensory (including pain) pathways • Deconditioning (e.g. lack of physical fitness in chronic fatigue, deconditioning of vestibular responsiveness in patients with dizziness who hold their head still) • Neuroendocrine and immunological abnormalities similar to those seen in depression and anxiety	• Perception of symptoms as being out with personal control/due to disease • Anxiety/ catastrophisation about cause of symptoms • Not being believed • Avoidance of symptom provocation (e.g. exercise in fatigue)	• Fear/avoidance of work or family responsibilities • The presence of a welfare system • Social benefits of being ill • Availability of legal compensation • Stigma of 'mental illness' in society and from medical profession

Source: Reproduced with permission from Stone J, Carson A, Sharpe M. Functional symptoms in neurology: management. *Journal of Neurology Neurosurgery and Psychiatry* 2005; 76(Suppl 1): i13–i21.

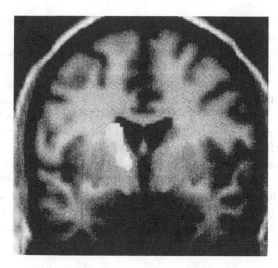

Figure 6.5 A composite scan of four patients with functional hemimotor and sensory symptoms compared to recovery. There was hypoactivation of the contralateral thalamus, caudate, and putamen during the symptomatic state

Source: Reproduced with permission from Vuilleumier P, Chicherio C, Assal F et al. Functional neuroanatomical correlates of hysterical sensorimotor loss. *Brain* 2001; 124: 1077–90.[21]

represent complex interplay of many variables. Many of the factors are similar for depression and anxiety.

When patients ask 'why has this happened?', the honest answer may be to say that you cannot be sure. This is the same response that one would give to a patient with migraine, multiple sclerosis or inflammatory bowel disease. One can certainly speculate about relevant predisposing factors but it probably wise for the clinician to remain aetiologically neutral with respect to the relative contribution of factors at the current time.

Rather than asking 'why has this happened', a more useful focus, certainly initially, is to discuss 'how has this happened'. This leads to more constructive discussion with the patient about how their nervous system may be 'going wrong' to produce the symptoms. Take the example of a patient who has a panic attack or physical injury, with marked depersonalisation followed by some residual weakness. It may be useful to consider what panic is, and how depersonalisation might persist abnormally, and how brain pathways may be affected, but it will be harder to be sure of why the person had the panic attack in the first place. Likewise, irritable bowel syndrome may be more common after infective diarrhoea, chronic fatigue syndrome after a fatiguing viral illness, and non-cardiac chest pain following a panic attack with chest tightness.

In contrast to precipitating factors, perhaps less emphasis is given than should be to perpetuating factors. This is of particular importance, as management of perpetuating factors may be most useful in patient treatment. Biologically, one must think both in terms of plasticity within the CNS, particularly involving pain pathways, but also of the effects on the rest of the body of altered behaviour such as deconditioning. Psychologically, there is an increasing body of evidence demonstrating that the cognitive beliefs held by a patient about their symptoms, in particular their own personal prediction of whether or not they will improve, or the cause of their symptoms, have a major effect on outcome.

Management

The range of presentations of unexplained symptoms is diverse, and clearly the approach to management needs to be tailored to the individual problems presented by the patient.[2,22]

Explanation

In our experience, an explanation of the diagnosis in positive terms is an absolutely essential stepping stone towards effective clinical management. This needs to be done in a way that is clear, logical, transparent and not offensive to the patient. It is surprising but it is this more than anything else that is often a major stumbling block to the clinician. In our experience, many clinicians simply do not know what to actually say to the patient and are bemused by which of the myriad of available terms is best to use. There is no single approach to explanation, but certain ways of saying things are, in our experience, more helpful than others.

We have advocated the use of the term functional symptoms for a number of reasons, both pragmatic and scientific. Thus, we might say to a patient that they have functional weakness as opposed to conversion disorder, hysterical or somatisation disorder. We believe that the advantages are that it replaces the erroneous physical versus psychological (brain/mind) debate and allows for a more productive discussion of whether the problem is functional (reversible) or structural (irreversible). Secondly, it provides a rationale for any treatment designed to

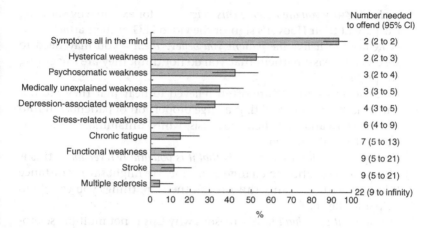

Figure 6.6 Diagnostic labels can be inherently offensive. The percentage of general neurology patients who equate the diagnosis with being 'mad', 'putting on' symptoms, or 'imagining symptoms', along with the number needed to offend – the number of patients that have to be given the diagnosis before one is offended; CI = confidence interval

Source: Reproduced with permission from Stone J, Wojcik W, Durrance D et al. What should we say to patients with symptoms unexplained by disease? The 'number needed to offend'. *BMJ* 2002; 325(7378): 1449–50.[23]

improve the function of the nervous system; in particular it allows for the use of both physical and psychological strategies. Thirdly, generally speaking, it avoids offence and allows transparency with the patient (Figure 6.6).[23] However, it is worth remembering that it is probably not the actual diagnostic label as much as the way in which it is explained and the attitude of the doctor approaching the consultation that are most important.

Many doctors simply explain to patients what they don't have; for example, a patient comes in with a weak leg and the doctor says it is 'okay there is no need to worry, you don't have multiple sclerosis'. Whilst this is generally pleasing news, what tends to be uppermost in the patient's mind is a desire to know what they *do* have and we suggest this should be the starting point of the explanation. In our experience, the most important elements in an explanation are:

1. *explaining what they do have* – for example, 'you have functional weakness', 'you have dissociative/non-epileptic attacks'
2. *explaining what this means in terms of 'mechanism'* – 'this occurs because your nervous system is not functioning properly'

3. *explaining why you are making this diagnosis* – for example by showing the patient their Hoover's sign or the video EEG of their attack
4. *being overt in telling the patient you believe them* – you may need to specifically reassure them that you do not think they are imagining the problem
5. *it's common* – patients are often relieved to hear that they are not particularly unusual and that a large proportion of patients fall into this category and that their diagnosis, whilst unfamiliar to them, is 'run of the mill' for you
6. *the implication of the diagnosis is that it is potentially reversible* – this is often a key cognition to change over time. We might say for instance 'I know you didn't bring this on, but there are things you can do to help it get better'
7. *explain what they don't have* – reasons why this is not multiple sclerosis, Crohn's disease, epilepsy etc
8. *usage of metaphors* – these obviously have to be adjusted to the social and cultural background of the patient that is being spoken to. Computer analogies such as 'the hardware is fine but the software has a glitch', or 'it is like a car/piano that is out of tune, all the parts are there they just aren't working right', can be helpful.

Some may criticise this approach as not being overtly psychological, or colluding with the patient. But our clinical experience is that an approach that does not force the issue of psychological aetiology paradoxically actually increases the subsequent emergence and discussion of relevant psychological symptoms and life problems. Our, possibly simplistic, understanding of this is that if the patient feels they have had a satisfactory assessment and sympathetic understanding of what they consider to be their primary problem, i.e. the weakness in their leg, they are then much more trusting of the doctor to raise issues that they have been much more guarded of up to that point in the consultation. One often finds, after this approach has been made, that the diagnosis is accepted and the patient will come back to you with a suggested psychological contribution to the aetiology, with a comment such as 'that is interesting doctor, certainly the symptoms came on at a point when I found out my husband was having an affair. Do you think that could be important?'. Clearly this information should be accepted and acted upon but again we would resist the temptation to use it as a whole explanation in a simple act of reattribution but rather try to view it as a piece of the jigsaw.

For any patient with mild symptoms, or early on in the presentation, a clear reassurance with encouragement to resume normal activities is frequently sufficient. For those patients with more resistant symptoms, the treatments described next may be helpful.

Physiotherapy/physical rehabilitation

Patients with physical problems often need physical treatments and certainly do appear to welcome them. It is our experience that high-quality physiotherapy with lots of explanation and encouragement to resume normal activity can have good results. There have been a number of encouraging case series of physical rehabilitation for patients with functional disability,[24] but unfortunately few have been randomised or report on very long-term outcome. Specifically looking at trials with chronic fatigue, there is now evidence at the level of systematic review that graded exercise is a helpful treatment.

Cognitive-behavioural therapy (CBT)

A review of cognitive-behavioural therapy (CBT) for all functional symptoms in 2000 showed that CBT can be effective across a wide range of functional somatic symptoms.[25] CBT emphasises the interaction between cognitive, behavioural, emotional and physiological factors in perpetuating symptoms. It aims to maximise function and reduce disability. It is conceived that the patient's cognitive interpretation of their bodily symptoms is key and that this will, in turn, depend upon their knowledge and experience of disease (Figure 6.7). CBT has a reputation for being rather mysterious but in fact many elements of it can be incorporated into most outpatient consultations:

- accept all symptoms at face value and give a positive explanation
- persuade the patient that change is possible, they are not damaged and they do have the potential to recover
- give the patient a rationale for treatment, for example, 'exercise will help recondition your muscles and tune up your nervous system'
- encourage activity in a graded fashion, warning the patient they may feel temporarily worse afterwards but there will be benefits in the long term
- counsel strongly against overdoing it on good days as much as underdoing it on bad days. Explain that symptoms tend to fluctuate and there will always be days where they feel back to square one
- encourage the setting of small achievable goals and gradual build-up
- establish a sleep routine. Give simple advice such as avoiding sleep during the day, getting up at a specified time, getting out of bed for 15 minutes rather than worrying awake at night

- encourage the patient to reconsider unhelpful and negative thoughts. For example, a patient with pain who thinks that walking will make the 'wear and tear' worse, should be encouraged to consider and test out an alternative possibility. That is, if they go for a walk they will be sore afterwards for a bit but in fact will be strengthening their bones and muscles and building confidence
- look for both physiological and dissociative trigger factors. If you can find evidence of dissociative symptoms before physical symptom onset, this will provide additional rationale for the type of treatment. For example, if a patient with non-epileptic attacks discloses such symptoms, a CBT approach similar to that used in panic, where patients are encouraged to be aware of catastrophic interpretation of symptoms and consider more benign ones, can be used
- look for obstacles to recovery. Rather than focusing on possible causes from the past, such as an unhappy childhood, focus on what is happening in the current day. This may include a hated job that they will have to return to, or a legal case that may not settle for 5 years. These issues can often be discussed openly and frankly and the patient encouraged to actively address them, once you have their trust. Where possible, provide more detailed written material.

As treatment progresses, it is usually possible to start making links between symptoms and stressful events. For example, 'when you had that terrible day what were you thinking about, what was happening, why might that have been relevant?'

Antidepressants and other drugs

Antidepressants can help many patients with functional symptoms, even those who are not depressed. A systematic review of antidepressant treatment in patients with a range of functional symptoms found a number needed to treat of three.[26] Of note, this review found the older tricyclic drugs had a stronger evidence base to support their use. This may in part have been artefactual as there were fewer trials of the more modern selective serotonin reuptake inhibitors (SSRIs), or it may have related to a greater effect of tricyclic drugs on pain. Importantly, analysis of the data suggested that the drugs were effective regardless of whether the patients were or were not clinically depressed.

In practice, patients are understandably suspicious of antidepressant drugs. Perceptions that they are addictive, harmful, just for mental illness, and have disabling side effects are widespread in the population. An open discussion about the pros and cons is important, emphasising

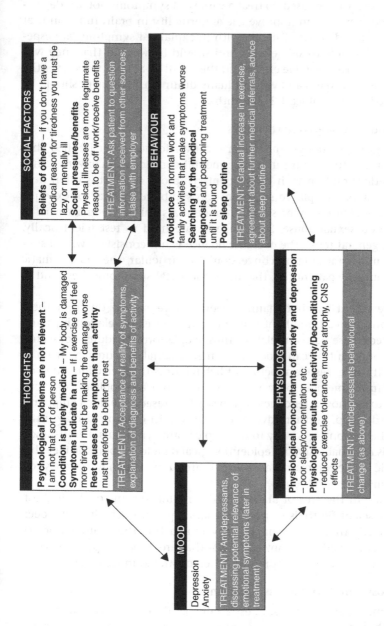

THOUGHTS

Psychological problems are not relevant –
I am not that sort of person
Condition is purely medical – My body is damaged
Symptoms indicate ha rm – If I exercise and feel
more tired I must be making the damage worse
Rest causes less symptoms than activity
must therefore be better be rest

TREATMENT: Acceptance of reality of symptoms,
explanation of diagnosis and benefits of activity

SOCIAL FACTORS

Beliefs of others – if you don't have a
medical reason for tiredness you must be
lazy or mentally ill
Social pressures/benefits
Physical illnesses are more legitimate
reason to be off work/receive benefits

TREATMENT: Ask patient to question
information received from other sources;
Liaise with employer

BEHAVIOUR

Avoidance of normal work and
family activities that make symptoms worse
**Searching for the medical
diagnoses** and postponing treatment
until it is found
Poor sleep routine

TREATMENT: Gradual increase in exercise,
agreement about further medical referrals, advice
about sleep routine

MOOD

Depression
Anxiety

TREATMENT: Antidepressants,
discussing potential relevance of
emotional symptoms (later in
treatment)

PHYSIOLOGY

Physiological concomitants of anxiety and depression
– poor sleep/concentration etc.
Physiological results of inactivity/Deconditioning
– reduced exercise tolerance, muscle atrophy, CNS
effects

TREATMENT: Antidepressants behavioural
change (as above)

Figure 6.7 A cognitive-behavioural model showing targets for treatment

Source: Reproduced with permission from Stone J, Carson A, Sharpe M. Functional symptoms in neurology: management. *Journal of Neurology Neurosurgery and Psychiatry* 2005; 76(Suppl 1): i13–i21.

that these are drugs used 'to treat a variety of symptoms not just depression and may help to improve the abnormality in brain function that we have talked about'. Patients with unexplained symptoms are especially vulnerable to side effects and should be warned that they will probably experience side effects but these will be at their worst over the first couple of weeks and will gradually diminish. Treatment should be persisted with for at least 2–3 months.

Psychodynamic psychotherapies

In classical psychodynamic theory, conversion disorder implied that distress resulting from intolerable mental conflict was converted into a somatic symptom with consequent symptom relief. It is often held that the actual displayed symptom was symbolic, so that for example a pseudo seizure may be said to represent a symbolic re-enactment of childhood sexual abuse. Such theories are hard to test scientifically, and in general terms the overall evidence is not consistent with a simplistic understanding of 'conversion'. In particular, the more somatic symptoms the patient has, the more emotional symptoms they tend to have.

More recent psychodynamic theories have moved on from these ideas and instead highlight the importance of early relationships and the effect these have on relationships people form as adults. For example, poor parenting can produce an interpersonal dependency in adulthood. If this excessive attachment behaviour is transferred to a doctor, or a family member only interested in physical problems, one can begin to see how a tendency to repeatedly present somatic complaints might develop. Further adverse experiences in childhood may influence the person's tendency to develop certain symptoms. For instance, there is reasonable quality epidemiological data to support the idea that chronic pelvic complaints are more common in women who were sexually abused in childhood.

In fact, in the area of unexplained symptoms, some of the highest-quality scientific trials of psychodynamic psychotherapies have been conducted. An interpersonal therapy approach to the treatment of irritable bowel syndrome showed results that are, broadly speaking, compatible with those more commonly demonstrated in CBT trials.[27]

Hypnosis and intravenous sedation

For some types of symptoms, especially paralysis and movement disorders, there may be a role for hypnosis or sedation as adjunctive treatments. In our own practice, we still use examination under sedation with a means to therapeutically demonstrate to the patient, with a video recording to look at afterwards, that apparently paralysed limbs can move, or fixed dystonic limbs are not in fact fixed. These techniques, however, are not treatments on their own, but rather are embedded within an overall rehabilitative framework and should only be attempted in patients with whom you have a good therapeutic relationship. We do not advocate attempting to gain further elements of the history using these techniques

The patient who does not get better

Many patients with these symptoms, despite having potentially reversible symptoms, have been ill for too long or have obstacles to recovery that are too powerful to overcome, even when they try. It is important for anyone attempting to treat this group of patients to realise this and know that there will be many times when a clinician may have to accept that there is nothing more they can do, even if the patient is very willing. At the present time, it is unclear whether we are being unduly pessimistic but bear in mind that, if one in three patients with chronic symptoms has a substantial improvement, then an attempt at treatment is worthwhile.

Conclusions

There is a growing realisation of the scale of the problem of patients with symptoms that are unexplained by disease. This is running in parallel with research challenging a purely psychological model of their causation. Patients with these symptoms can be time consuming to assess but potentially very rewarding if they improve. We have tried to provide a very practical approach to assessment and management that is, in part, evidence based, although there remains much to find out.

Key learning points

- Patients with symptoms unexplained by disease are common, frequently have depression and anxiety, and have self-reported disability comparable to patients with disease.
- As long as the patient is assessed by a competent physician, the diagnosis, at least in neurology, is as accurate as any other disease diagnosis (about 5% diagnostic change at 5 years).
- 'Psychiatric' terminology may be misinterpreted as offensive by patients and care should be taken with language and attitude.

A diagnosis of neurological symptoms unexplained by disease should only be made using positive signs. Familiarity with these signs helps with psychiatric assessment and explanation.

Initial explanations of symptoms work best when describing 'what' the problem is and the potential physiological mechanism of the symptoms, rather than attempting to explain physical symptoms purely in terms of previous life events or psychological states.

When trying to help a patient with chronic symptoms, only expect some to get better. Do not blame yourself or the patient if they do not.

Key references

Hallett M, Cloninger CR, Fahn S, Jankovic J, Lang AE, Yudofsky SC. *Psychogenic Movement Disorders*. Philadelphia: Lippincott Williams and Wilkins and the American Academy of Neurology; 2005.

Halligan P, Bass C, Marshall JC. *Contemporary Approaches to the Science Of Hysteria: Clinical and Theoretical Perspectives*. Oxford: Oxford University Press; 2001.

Halligan PW, Bass C, Oakley DA. *Malingering and Illness Deception*. Oxford: Oxford University Press; 2003.

Lloyd GG, Guthrie E. *Handbook of Liaison Psychiatry*. Cambridge: Cambridge University Press; 2007.

Mayou R, Sharpe M, Carson A. *ABC of Psychological Medicine*. London:: BMJ Publishing Group; 2003.

Wessely S, Hotopf M, Sharpe M. *Chronic Fatigue and its Syndromes*. Oxford: Oxford University Press; 1998.

References

1. Stone J, Carson A, Sharpe M. Functional symptoms and signs in neurology: assessment and diagnosis. *Journal of Neurology Neurosurgery and Psychiatry* 2005; 76(Suppl 1): i–i12.

2. Stone J, Carson A, Sharpe M. Functional symptoms in neurology: management. *Journal of Neurology Neurosurgery and Psychiatry* 2005; 76(Suppl 1): i13–i21.

3. Deyo RA, Weinstein JN. Low back pain. *New England Journal of Medicine* 2001; 344(5): 363–70.

4. Robins LN, Helzer JE, Weissman MM , Orvaschel H; Gruenberg E; Burke Jr JD; Regier DA Lifetime prevalence of specific psychiatric disorders in three sites. *Archives of General Psychiatry* 1984; 41(10): 949–58.

5. Gureje O, Simon GE, Ustun TB, Goldberg DP. Somatization in cross-cultural perspective: a World Health Organization study in primary care. *American Journal of Psychiatry* 1997; 154(7): 989–95.

6. Kroenke K, Mangelsdorff AD. Common symptoms in ambulatory care: incidence, evaluation, therapy, and outcome. *American Journal of Medicine* 1989; 86(3): 262–6.

7. Perkin GD. An analysis of 7836 successive new outpatient referrals. *Journal of Neurology Neurosurgery and Psychiatry* 1989; 52(4): 447–8.
8. Binzer M, Andersen PM, Kullgren G. Clinical characteristics of patients with motor disability due to conversion disorder: a prospective control group study. *Journal of Neurology Neurosurgery and Psychiatry* 1997; 63(1): 83–8.
9. Reuber M, Elger CE. Psychogenic nonepileptic seizures: review and update. *Epilepsy and Behaviour* 2003; 4(3): 205–16 Stone J, Smyth R, Carson A , Lewis S, Prescott R, Warlow C, Sharpe M. Systematic review of misdiagnosis of conversion symptoms and 'hysteria'. *BMJ* 2005; 331(7523): 989.
10. Slater ET. Diagnosis of 'hysteria'. *British Medical Journal* 1965; i: 1395–1399.
11. Ron M. The prognosis of hysteria / somatisation disorder. In: Halligan P, Bass C, Marshall JC, editors. *Contemporary Approaches to the Study of Hysteria*. Oxford: Oxford University Press; 2001, p. 271–81.
12. Hadler NM. If You Have to Prove You Are Ill, You Can't Get Well: The Object Lesson of Fibromyalgia. *Spine Volume* 21(20), 2397–2400.
13. Schilte AF, Portegijs PJ, Blankenstein AH van der Horst HE, Latour MBF, van Eijk JTM, Knottnerus JA. Randomised controlled trial of disclosure of emotionally important events in somatisation in primary care. *BMJ* 2001; 323(7304): 86.
14. Stone J, Smyth R, Carson A, Warlow C, Sharpe M. La belle indifference in conversion symptoms and hysteria: systematic review. *British Journal of Psychiatry* 2006; 188: 204–209.
15. Hallett M, Fahn S, Jankovic J, Lang AE, Cloninger CR, Yudofski SC. *Psychogenic Movement Disorders*. Philadelphia: Lippincott Williams and Wilkins and the American Academy of Neurology; 2005.
16. Charcot JM. *Clinical Lectures on Diseases of the Nervous System* (Volume 3). London: New Sydenham Society; 1889.
17. Kim YJ, Pakiam AS, Lang AE. Historical and clinical features of psychogenic tremor: a review of 70 cases. *Canadian Journal of Neurological Science* 1999; 26(3): 190–5.
18. Schrag A, Trimble M, Quinn N, Bhatia K. The syndrome of fixed dystonia: an evaluation of 103 patients. *Brain* 2004; 127(10): 2360–72.
19. Lempert T, Brandt T, Dieterich M, Huppert D. How to identify psychogenic disorders of stance and gait. A video study in 37 patients. *Journal of Neurology* 1991; 238(3): 140–6.
20. Waddell G. *The Back Pain Revolution*. Edinburgh: Churchill Livingstone; 2004.
21. Vuilleumier P, Chicherio C, Assal F Schwartz S, Slosman D, Landis T. Functional neuroanatomical correlates of hysterical sensorimotor loss. *Brain* 2001; 124: 1077–90.
22. Henningsen P, Zipfel S, Herzog W. Management of functional somatic syndromes. *Lancet* 2007; 369(9565): 946–55.
23. Stone J, Wojcik W, Durrance D Carson A, Lewis S, Mackenzie L, Warlow CP, Sharpe M. What should we say to patients with symptoms unexplained by disease? The 'number needed to offend'. *BMJ* 2002; 325(7378): 1449–50.
24. Wade D. Rehabilitation for conversion symptoms. In: Halligan P, Bass C, Marshall JC, editors. *Contemporary Approaches to the Study of Hysteria*. Oxford: Oxford University Press; 2001, p. 330–46.

128   *Alan Carson and Jon Stone*

25. Kroenke K, Swindle R. Cognitive-behavioral therapy for somatization and symptom syndromes: a critical review of controlled clinical trials. *Psychotherapy and Psychosomatics* 2000; 69(4): 205–15.
26. O'Malley PG, Jackson JL, Santoro J, Tomkins G, Balden E, Kroenke K. Antidepressant therapy for unexplained symptoms and symptom syndromes. *Journal of Family Practice* 1999; 48(12): 980–90.
27. Guthrie E, Creed F, Dawson D, Tomenson B. A randomised controlled trial of psychotherapy in patients with refractory irritable bowel syndrome. *British Journal of Psychiatry* 1993; 163: 315–21.

7

Psychological Conceptualisation and Treatment Approaches to Functional Non-Epileptic Attacks

Danielle Gaynor and Niruj Agrawal

Functional non-epileptic attacks (FNEA) are involuntary, paroxysmal changes in sensory/motor activity and/or consciousness, without the encephalographic (EEG) changes typical of epileptic attacks. They do not arise from the specific central nervous system (CNS) dysfunctions underlying epilepsy. Non-epileptic seizures may be of organic or non-organic types. Organic types (10–20%) may result from head injury, ischaemic attacks, narcolepsy, hemiplegic migraine, paroxysmal vertigo, cardiac arrhythmia, hypoglycaemia or syncope.[1] Non-organic FNEA, on the other hand, are psychogenic in nature (80–90%), having no physiological aetiology.

It is important to emphasise that while non-organic in nature, these attacks are real, and can have devastating personal, social and economic impact. Many FNEA patients have poor social functioning, and are unable to hold down a job. FNEA represents a considerable drain on family or public resources. Patients' repeated visits to emergency and other medical services run at an estimated annual cost of $110–920 million.[2] FNEA patients score low on quality-of-life scales and their health-related quality of life is rated even lower than that of patients with refractory epilepsy.[3] They describe a significantly poorer profile of perceived health status compared with patients with epilepsy.

Unfortunately, diagnostic delays of years are still a rule rather than an exception. Most patients are treated for years as suffering from epilepsy, with several antiepileptic drugs. Many patients with FNEA have a tendency to seek medical attention frequently. A significant proportion will present as status epilepticus and quarter to half of all admissions to neurology intensive therapy unit (ITU) departments are found to have non-epileptic status.

Terminology

FNEAs have been known as 'hysterical seizures', 'pseudoseizures', 'psychogenic seizures', 'non-epileptic seizures', 'non-epileptic attack disorder (NEAD)', 'psychogenic non-epileptic seizures (PNES)' or 'dissociative convulsions', to name a few. Some of these names, such as 'hysterical seizures' and 'pseudoseizures', are considered to be unsatisfactory because they are pejorative, and so have been largely abandoned. Other terms such as non-epileptic seizures and NEAD are considered unsatisfactory on the grounds that they merely describe what the patient hasn't got rather than describing the condition the patient suffers from. These terms also do not differentiate between organic causes and psychogenic causes of non-epileptic fits. However, a number of these terminologies remain in common use, particularly FNEA, PNES and NEAD. There is considerable ongoing debate about what this disorder should be called, perpetuating inconsistent use of terminology. We prefer FNEA to describe this condition and will use it in this chapter.

Epidemiology

The prevalence of FNEA has been estimated to be 5–20% of the outpatient epilepsy population. Rates as high as 25–30% have been reported in tertiary clinic patients referred for refractory epilepsy.[4] Data from population studies show an incidence rate of 3–4.6 per 100,000 population and a prevalence of 2–33 per 100,000 of the general population.[5] Data from Iceland similarly show the incidence of FNEA to be 5% of that of epilepsy.[6] Although prevalence figures are not given, FNEA case reports come from around the world.[7–11]

Between 75% and 80% of FNEA patients are females and though fewer men with this condition may be seeking help, there is still a high likelihood of clear female preponderance. Most patients with FNEA have their first episode in early adulthood and it is rare in children under 10 years of age. This condition is known to occur in older adults. FNEA are thought to be more common in people with lower educational[12] and socio-economic background.

Clinical presentation and diagnosis

Diagnosis of epilepsy and FNEA remains essentially clinical. Careful history taking from the patient and a close family member who has seen a fit is essential for differential diagnosis. The sequence of events before, during and after a fit should be established, including the duration of various phases. It is often helpful to gain information about the initial fit, stressful life events surrounding the fit (if present), subsequent investigation, diagnosis and progression.

Attempts should be made first of all to differentiate epileptic attacks from non-epileptic attacks and to subsequently differentiate organic non-epileptic attacks from FNEA. Common causes of organic non-epileptic attacks should be considered and ruled out (Table 7.1). There is no single diagnostic factor in the history or examination but a number of factors may point towards a non-epileptic cause or psychogenic nature of the fits.

Clinical features that are traditionally considered manifestations of epileptic seizures, such as tongue biting, incontinence, stereotyped attacks, injury, frothing, apparent progression from aura to fit to a post-ictal stage, etc. can be commonly seen in FNEA. Features that are suggestive of FNEA are described in Box 7.1. No single clinical or historical feature is diagnostic of epilepsy or FNEA. However, as the number of unusual features for epilepsy increases, FNEA should be considered.

Past medical and psychiatric history, personal history and premorbid personality characteristics can help in the diagnosis. Past presentations with multiple unexplained somatic symptoms, history of psychiatric illnesses and treatment can help with the diagnosis. Past traumatic events, including childhood sexual abuse, have been linked with FNEA.

Table 7.1 Common causes of non-epileptic attacks

Organic	Functional (FNEA)
• Syncope	• Panic disorders
• Hyperventilation	• Depersonalisation disorder
• Transient ischaemic attacks	• Hypochondriasis
• Paroxysmal movement disorders	• Somatisation disorder
• Narcolepsy	• Dissociative/conversion disorders
• Non-epileptic myoclonus	• Depressive disorder
• Hypoglycaemia	• Post-traumatic stress disorder (PTSD)
• Myasthenia gravis	• Factitious disorders

Box 7.1 Clinical features suggestive of FNEA

Prolonged duration of seizures (>2 minutes)
Fluctuating course
Gradual onset (slow increase of symptoms)
Asynchronous movements
Side-to-side head movement
Out-of-phase limb movements
Thrashing movement of entire body
Unresponsiveness without motor movements
Recall for period of unresponsiveness.
Resistance to eye opening
Pelvic thrusting
Opisthotonus
Jaw clenching in tonic phase
Variability of symptoms
Planter and corneal reflex normal
High degree of affect in vocalisations
Weeping

Non-epileptic fits can present in various ways. Box 7.2 describes some of the more common presentations of FNEA, which may occur in isolation or in combination.

New methods of correctly differentiating between epilepsy and FNEA include the use of conversational analysis of the patient's description of their fits.[13] Recognition of stertorous breathing has been similarly described as useful.[14] These findings may help to improve the reliability of clinical diagnosis in the future.

The gold standard for diagnosis remains long video-EEG telemetry if it captures a typical fit. However, this is expensive and still not readily available at all centres. A good-quality home video can be equally useful in confirming the clinical diagnosis. A single inter-ictal EEG may not contribute to diagnosis and may be normal. Conversely, abnormal EEGs can be found in over half of patients with FNEA. Some patients may even show epileptiform abnormalities. Absence of post-ictal EEG changes may be a more reliable predictor of FNEA.

Provocation procedures such as hyperventilation and photic stimulation are commonly used with EEG to increase the likelihood of capturing a seizure during EEG. Some clinicians advocate the use of provocation procedures, such as saline infusion, suggestion, application of alcohol pads or a tuning fork to the patient's head, etc during video-EEG telemetry, to increase the chances of capturing a seizure. Other clinicians express ethical concerns about such practices and feel that

Box 7.2   Common clinical presentations of FNEA

● *Panic attacks* – these may resemble epileptic seizures and loss of consciousness may occur
● *Avoidance attacks (swoons)* – typically these occur when one is unable to cope with a stressful situation, and individuals may fall to the floor and remain inert with reduced muscle tone
● *Abreactive attacks* – these occur as a delayed response to highly stressful experiences, and often occur towards the latter part of the day. Hyperventilation may precede increased body tone and thrashing of the limbs
● *Simulated attacks* – conscious or unconscious simulation of an epileptic seizure, usually involving some kind of gain

it can affect the doctor–patient relationship and may not be acceptable to patients.

Additional investigations such as serum prolactin levels within 20 minutes of seizures have gone out of favour due to poor sensitivity and specificity. Similarly, the use of brain scans is non-contributory in reaching a correct diagnosis.

Frontal lobe seizures are most likely to be misdiagnosed with FNEA as they are often associated with normal scalp EEG and video-EEG telemetry. Moreover, they are likely to present with some of the clinical features suggestive of FNEA. Usually, features such as very short duration, onset during sleep and stereotypical nature help with correct diagnosis.

Psychiatric classification and comorbidities

The *Diagnostic and Statistical Manual of Mental Disorders* (4th edition, text revision; DSM-IV-TR)[15] classifies FNEA as a subtype of conversion disorder within the group of somatoform disorders, whereas the *International Statistical Classification of Diseases and Related Health Problems* (10th edition; ICD-10)[16] classifies FNEA as dissociative seizures within the broad category of dissociative disorders, which subsumes all the conversion disorders.

FNEA may be further classified according to subtype, according to the psychiatric condition either comorbid with, or triggering, the attacks. FNEA patients are commonly seen to be suffering from depression, anxiety disorders (including PTSD), or dissociation. The demarcation between these conditions, however, may not be so clear cut, nor is comorbidity limited to these three. Moreover, in an FNEA patient sample,[17] the mean number of current axis 1 psychiatric diagnoses was 4.4. This is consistent with findings by Mökleby.[18] Not all FNEA patients, however, have psychiatric comorbity. Jawad et al. found no psychiatric disorder in 32.6% of their FNEA population sample screened using the structured clinical interview for the DSM-IIIR.[19]

Depression has been seen to occur in 12–57% of patients.[20] Roy and Barris documented 100% of their FNEA patient sample as being depressed.[21] While some of these cases may be classified as dysthymic disorder, Bowman and Markand found up to 47% of FNEA patients report current major depression,[17] while 50–80% of patients report past episodes of major depression. Because of these high levels of comorbidity, it is recommended that all FNEA patients be screened for depression.

Anxiety disorders, including post-traumatic stress disorder (PTSD), are also extremely common amongst FNEA patients, being seen in 10–47% of FNEA cases.[17,19] Moreover, the frightening nature of the seizures themselves is also a source of considerable stress. High proportions of FNEA patients have also been reported to have traumatic histories.[17]

Traumatic experiences, such as war or other disasters, or sexual, physical or emotional abuse, may often also account for the dissociative disorder comorbidity which is reported in 10%[19] to 90%[17] of FNEA patients. Mean scores of FNEA patients on the dissociative experience scale were significantly higher than those of epilepsy patients or patients with both types of seizures.[22] Bowman describes dissociation as the 'mechanism of action of conversion disorders' involving alterations in consciousness and memory by splitting off of some aspects of experience from consciousness, creating two or more parallel, concurrent systems of awareness within the mind.[23] One system may be available to everyday consciousness, whilst another system may convert traumatic or otherwise unacceptable experiential content into physical symptoms. These symptoms often express dissociated emotions (anger, fear, sadness) or psychological conflicts (e.g. between love and hate for the abusive parent), or may represent a behavioural reliving of traumatic experiences (reliving combat whilst in a state of amnesia). Pelvic thrusting in a victim of sexual abuse is considered to be an example of dissociated mental content expressed though FNEA. Other somatoform disorders (e.g. somatoform pain, numbness, blindness and other visual disturbances, deafness, fainting) are also common in this patient group.

Personality disorders (paranoid, borderline, avoidant, and histrionic) have also been flagged up in correlation with FNEA. Personality profiling using the Minnesota Multiphasic Personality Inventory (MMPI) and MMPI-2 has shown FNEA patients have high scores on the hysteria, hypochondriasis, depression and schizophrenia scales. The most common profiles were conversion and somatoform disorders; however, dysthymic and depressive patterns were also seen. Thus, FNEA patients are not seen to form a homogeneous group.[24,25]

Moreover, FNEA may in fact be misdiagnosed panic attacks, dissociative trance episodes, or flashbacks of trauma.[23]. In these cases, FNEA are better diagnosed as panic disorder, dissociative disorder not otherwise specified, or PTSD. Others have proposed alternative classification systems for FNEA.[26–28] This lack of consensus is further reflected in the difference in the way current classification manuals such as the DSM-IV and the ICD-10 categorise FNEA.

Aetiologies and triggers

Depression, anxiety disorders, and dissociative disorders are all responses to life stresses, as indeed are FNEA episodes themselves. For this reason, some conceive of FNEA as 'stress-related seizures'.[29] It is this commonality that makes it so difficult to draw clear distinctions between FNEA subtypes. The picture is further complicated in that identical circumstances will elicit different responses in different individuals. Reactive predispositions have been ascribed to neuronal development in early childhood, which link to attachment processes with the child's primary carer.[30]

The aetiology of FNEA remains ambiguous, however, with the precise mental processes leading to seizures as yet unidentified. Numerous studies indicate a high correlation with childhood and adolescent sexual, psychological and physical abuse.[31,32] This has been replicated,[33] although the large-sample study indicates that childhood psychological abuse is the only unique predictor of FNEA when comparing FNEA to epilepsy patients. One implication of this is that the emphasis on the aetiological role of sexual abuse may be an oversimplification, and could potentially divert clinical concern from other more important causal factors.

An aetiological scheme that describes potential predisposing factors, precipitating factors and perpetuating factors remains, in our view, the clinically most useful approach to understanding the roles of various aetiological factors (Box 7.3).

Box 7.3   Aetiological factors for FNEA

Predisposing factors

Sexual or physical abuse
Premorbid personality
Shaping factor such as symptom modelling
Somatoform/conversion/dissociative disorders

Precipitating factors

Acute stress
Life events
Acute psychiatric conditions (e.g. panic disorder)

Perpetuating factors

Maladaptive coping strategy
Adoption of sick role
Secondary gains
Intentional or unintentional reinforcements

Applying therapeutic models

An important and recurrent theme in the FNEA literature is that the choice of therapeutic procedure should depend upon the underlying, or comorbid, psychopathology. Many approaches have been applied, including cognitive-behavioural, cognitive, behavioural, psychodynamic and family therapy, hypnosis and psychopharmacological therapy. Numerous case studies, case series and open trials of these treatment modalities have been reported, and provide the beginnings of an empirical foundation to guide treatment (see Gaynor, Cock and Agrawal for a systematic review of the evidence base).[34]

Although there is good evidence that merely presenting the diagnosis in a sensitive and educative manner may lead to cessation of attacks in a number of patients,[35] the majority of patients are referred for psychotherapy. At the time of writing, only one randomised controlled trial (RCT) of a specific treatment approach has been completed.[36] This study showed paradoxical therapy to be more effective than anxiolytics in the management of FNEA. However, given the small sample sizes and the fact that treatment conditions between the two groups differed in other important ways, further investigation of this approach is warranted. Moreover, it is difficult, if not impossible, to evaluate any approach independently of other overlapping or concurrent therapeutic influences. The environmental and intrapsychic triggers of seizures are also often complex and multidimensional, so that treatment programmes are frequently designed to attack more than one single problem. Reports of therapeutic interventions tend to group approaches into categories. However, these distinctions generally reflect different theoretical orientations rather than mutually exclusive or rigorously operational differences in actual work with patients.

The cognitive-behavioural perspective sees FNEA as dissociative responses to fear and anxiety engendered by intolerable or fearful circumstances. Thus, seizures may be understood in terms of a 'fear-avoidance' model. Seizure behaviour is perpetuated by a vicious circle of cognitive, behavioural, affective, physiological and social factors. Among these, the fear–avoidance dyad plays a prominent role. Fear of new seizures leads the patient to modify or avoid certain activities, behaviours or situations. Avoidance is counterproductive, however, as it focuses attention on the possibility of further seizures. Avoidance increases fear of seizures, while doing nothing to actually prevent them. Within the framework of the 'fear avoidance' model, standard cognitive-behavioural therapy (CBT) interventions such as desensitisation and graded exposure to feared stimuli, problem solving and anxiety management may be used as treatment of dissociative symptoms. CBT approaches can be used to identify and control factors that precipitate and maintain dissociative seizures. Less demanding than psychoanalytic approaches, CBT has been found to be effective in many individual cases reviewed.[37] Goldstein et al. piloted a CBT trial, with 81% of their patient sample showing at least a partial reduction in attacks at 6-month follow-up.[38] More recently, LaFrance et al. reported that 65% of their patients were attack free at the end of their open trial of manualised CBT.[39] Improvements were also seen on measures of depression, anxiety, somatic symptoms, quality of life and psychosocial functioning.

Cognitive and behavioural techniques have been recommended for anxiety-related FNEA.[40] This is consistent with Ettinger et al.,[41] who found that pending litigation was a predictive factor for poor FNEA prognosis. Litigation is likely to be associated with increased stress levels, which may in turn lead to increased FNEA.

Unexplained dissociative and somatic conditions, such as FNEA, may also be conceived as 'cognitive dysfunctional disorders'. From a cognitive perspective, the function of dissociation is to protect the individual from overwhelming affect. It is speculated that somatic symptoms may be symbolic representations of the original conflict itself.[42] This draws on Janet's suggestion that the effects of trauma result in a disconnection of experience and its behavioural response from consciousness. Focusing on higher- and lower-level attentional systems, Brown expanded Janet's ideas into his own cognitive conceptual model.[43] This model holds that many routine, apparently automatic, behaviours (requiring low levels of attention) may be associated with emotions and beliefs derived from the surrounding environment. These are then influenced by primary (e.g. emotional) and secondary (e.g. financial) gain, in ways that feel and appear involuntary. It is these 'automatic' behaviours that become the focus of the therapeutic intervention. Treatment would involve raising the patient's awareness of these behaviours and their associated distorted cognitions, with the goal of changing the cognitions and the behaviours they drive.

As with the cognitive-behavioural or cognitive perspectives, the behavioural point of view is that FNEA are maladaptive dissociative responses to difficult or unpleasant emotions or situations. The behaviouralists' specificity is their focus on the reinforcement of these responses through attention from family, physicians and other carers.[44] Operant conditioning has been reported to be effective for patients with low IQ,[45] or cognitive impairments,[46,47] as well as for children. Alsaadi and Marquez review the use of behavioural techniques for patients with PTSD and dissociation, as well as for those with reinforced behaviour patterns.[48] Operant conditioning appears to be helpful in FNEA cases where secondary gain seems to be an important maintaining factor.[59,49,50]

Psychodynamic approaches may also be chosen when underlying difficulties involve interpersonal difficulties and/or unresolved emotional conflicts, especially those pertaining to early abuse or other childhood traumas.[65] This follows Freud's view that incestuous sexual abuse creates an association between sex drives and fear, guilt and shame, resulting in a conflict between innate sexual drives and the aversive feelings with which they have become associated.[51] This painful conflict is then excluded from conscious awareness, leading to its expression as somatic complaints (conversion). LaFrance and Barry[42] stress that the primary focus of psychodynamic therapy is to examine the role of trauma and dissociation, inadequate attachment, and the patient's difficulty in coping with intrapsychic conflict and anxiety. The importance of stressful relationships and events, which are often instrumental in the development of FNEA as a coping strategy, is also emphasised.[51] Bowman[23] and Reuber and House[52] concur that intensive psychotherapy may help patients to acknowledge, accept and express threatening emotions and to develop realistic, attainable expectations for themselves and others. This can be useful for patients with more severe forms of emotional disorder associated with affect deregulation and deficient interpersonal skills (e.g. borderline personality disorder).

Family or relationship dysfunction has been much discussed as a predisposing, precipitating and/or perpetuating factor for many psychiatric disorders, including FNEA,[31,33] and it is argued that severe or chronic stress is a common element to all aetiological factors for FNEA, particularly when patients are not buffered by secure and loving family relationships.[53] Poor family functioning and denial may delay long-term recovery. These factors are also frequently associated with relapse.[54] In a study of families of children with FNEA, two broad patterns were identified: disorganised, chaotic families, and those that are anxious and preoccupied with disease.[55] Another study showed that compared to epilepsy patients and healthy controls, FNEA patients see their family members as less committed to and supportive of each other.[56] This initial finding may support a role for family involvement in the treatment of FNEA patients, as well as potentially leading to better understanding of the aetiology of the disorder.

It has also been suggested that illness may provide an escape from everyday problems and offer the family an acceptable excuse for disappointments and lack of success.[57] Moreover, in the face of illness, inadequate communication and unfair reward/punishment systems become less important and may be temporarily put aside. Thus, somatisation may help to consolidate the family. However, such behaviours usually have a long history, sometimes spanning generations. True motivations for these behaviours are therefore rarely obvious, making therapy more difficult.

Although the primary target for therapeutic benefit is the patient, family or systemic interventions also aim to lower stress levels and improve functioning of members of the patient's entourage. This need is illustrated in findings that family members are often also highly anxious, and may also be angry about the diagnosis.[75] Moreover, protectiveness may lead them to severely restrict the patient's activities and autonomy so that the patient is never left alone. Education and reassurance of family members aims to lower the family's anxiety levels. This may have positive knock-on effects for the patients, thus reinforcing the direct benefits of the intervention for the patient. Involving families and recruiting their support may help to reduce resistance to individual talking therapies.[23] Moreover, family interventions can be combined with individual therapy for adults, in order to reinforce better coping mechanisms, as well as to help the family to stop reinforcing FNEA symptoms. This is most frequently helpful with children and adolescents, as has been found by several studies.[58,59]

One characteristic feature of FNEA is that in many patients they may be triggered or halted by suggestion. This has been exploited in the diagnostic process, as well as in treatment, dating back to Charcot and Freud.[27] A review of the growing body of literature on the treatment of FNEA found two small studies, of poor methodological quality, that assessed hypnosis. Unfortunately, neither of these trials provides reliable evidence for the benefits of this type of intervention. Another study, using a structured questionnaire with 20 patients to investigate levels of dissociation, escape-avoidance coping strategies and hypnotisability did not show elevated hypnotisability in FNEA patients,[60] in contrast to findings by Kuyk et al.[61] This is somewhat surprising, given reports of neuroimaging data that confirm that conversion symptoms and hypnosis involve common neurological pathways.[62] It is suggested that hypnosis may be a valuable adjunct to other therapies, but that it is not essential for improvement.[69] Moreover, while hypnosis on its own may improve conversion symptoms, it may have no impact upon the underlying psychopathology. For this reason, a comprehensive approach may be more effective.

In practice, strict demarcation between the theoretical bases for the different psychological approaches is not always maintained. The underlying psychodynamic features vary widely between one patient and another, and often require multiple, simultaneous therapeutic approaches.[63] Moreover, numerous clinicians have combined individual treatments with group programmes, such as individual CBT or psychodynamic therapies with group psycho-education.[64] These combinations have the unfortunate downside of making controlled trials of specific techniques difficult, if not impossible. However, there is empirical support for the use of a mixture of treatment modalities.[65,66]

Behaviour therapy has been reported to be associated with complete recovery in the case of a 13-year-old girl who had become subject to sudden falls.[67] Cognitive techniques supported by pharmacology were recommended as adjuncts to address her comorbid obsessive-compulsive disorder, and poor insight.

A five-year study followed 128 patients with FNEA who were offered operant conditioning; anxiety management; abreaction; psychotherapy or counselling; family therapy; and psychopharmacology (major tranquilisers), either in combination or alone.[68] Complete attack resolution was seen in 63% of patients at discharge (31% at 5-year follow-up), partial resolution in 24% of cases (14% at follow-up), no change or worse for 13% (and 34% five years later). The authors do not report whether mixing approaches was more effective than the use of single-approach treatments. Positive results were also reported in another study whose subjects crucially reported improvements in social functioning and reduced demands on healthcare services.[69]

Not all FNEA patients, however, accept the psychological aetiology of their condition, and may be offended by, or reluctant to accept, a referral for psychotherapy. In cases where patients decline talking therapies, pharmacological treatments have been used. Medication may also be used as an adjunct to psychotherapy. First, however, numerous authors recommend withdrawing patients from antiepileptic drugs, unless they suffer from comorbid epilepsy.[47] There is further anecdotal support for the use of selective serotonin reuptake inhibitors (SSRIs), beta-blockers, analgesics and benzodiazepines to provide relief from some of the comorbid or underlying psychopathologies.[70] The use of benzodiazepines in treatment of comorbid or underlying anxiety should be avoided because they risk addiction without treating and solving the underlying problem.[23] These medications should be used as last-resort treatments for patients who refuse talking therapies.

Outcomes

The outcome for FNEA patients is generally considered to be poor. Short-term attack reduction and cessation rates as high as 50%[38] and 81%[71] have been seen. However, corresponding improvements in psychosocial functioning do not necessarily follow. Ettinger et al. report that at a mean of 18 months following diagnosis, 56 patients responded to a telephone-based questionnaire.[72] During that time, 53.6% of patients (including 44.8% of those whose FNEA had resolved) had been rehospitalised for FNEA or other symptoms, including depression, suicidal ideation and suicide attempts, and only patients whose seizures had resolved were employed. Factors most highly associated with seizure resolution were belief in the FNEA diagnosis, and improved health, occupational, and family functioning, but these were found only in 69%, 48% and 48% respectively of resolved seizure cases.

Longer-term outcomes have also been examined in several studies. At five or more years after diagnosis,[73] only 29% of one patient sample was free from FNEA (with no other conversion symptoms) and 15% had occasional seizures; 35% of the patients, however, still suffered from psychological or physical conditions causing functional difficulties, but not complete disability. The remaining 21% were considered to have a 'very poor' outcome, which indicated near or complete incapacitation or death. Although FNEA were the major cause of difficulty in only

5% of cases, psychosocial problems continued in 55%, with other psychological disturbances taking precedence. This pattern has been confirmed in subsequent studies.[74] Reuber et al. likewise found that 71.2% of patients continued to have seizures 4 years after diagnosis, and that 56.4% depended on health-dependent state benefits for their living.[75] They also found better outcome to be associated with younger onset and diagnosis, attacks with less-dramatic features, fewer comorbid somatic complaints, lower dissociation scores, and higher levels of education. Seizure remission may not be the most important outcome measure and certainly is not the only outcome measure. The focus should also be on overall functioning, quality of life, independent living and reduction in help-seeking behaviour.

Conclusions

FNEA are a highly complex psychogenic expression of subconscious emotional distress, affecting 5% to 20% of patients seen in specialist epilepsy clinics around the world, and 2 to 33 per 100,000 of the general population. Patients generally have poor social and occupational functioning, and represent a considerable drain on family, state and medical resources.

These attacks are seen to arise from, or accompany, a variety of psychiatric disorders, in particular depression, anxiety disorders and dissociative disorders. Traumatic events, as well as severe and chronic family or life stresses, are frequently seen as aetiological factors. Interventions covering the range of psychotherapeutic approaches have been used in the treatment of FNEA, although only one RCT testing any specific approach has been completed to date. Anecdotal evidence suggests that treatment should be based upon the underlying or comorbid psychopathology, and tailored to the specific circumstances of the individual patient. However, early diagnosis and tactful presentation of the diagnosis to the patient, along with psycho-education, remains the essential prerequisite for good eventual outcome. There remains a need for further treatment research. However, because of the complex environmental and intrapsychic interactions, it will be difficult, if not impossible, to evaluate individual therapeutic influences.

Key learning points

● FNEA are involuntary, paroxysmal changes in sensory/motor activity and/or consciousness but do not arise from the central nervous system dysfunction underlying epilepsy. The vast majority of these are psychogenic in origin.

FNEA are commonly seen (up to one-third of patients) in epilepsy clinics. Approximately one-third of FNEA patients can have both epileptic and non-epileptic fits.

No single diagnostic factor in the examination or history is diagnostic of epilepsy or FNEA. As the number of unusual features for epilepsy increases, a diagnosis of FNEA should be considered. The gold standard for FNEA diagnosis remains video-EEG telemetry, if it captures a typical fit. Early accurate diagnosis and appropriate presentation of diagnosis to the patient determines the prognosis. The choice of psychological treatment modality is often influenced by underlying or comorbid psychiatric conditions (e.g. anxiety, depression or dissociative disorders). Treatment approaches should be individually tailored and may be combined to address more than one issue.

Key references

Bowman ES, Markand ON. Psychodynamics and psychiatric diagnoses of pseudoseizure subjects. *American Journal of Psychiatry* 1996; 153: 57–63.

Ettinger AB, Devinsky O, Weisbrot DM, Ramakrishna RK, Goyal A. A comprehensive profile of clinical, psychiatric, and psychosocial characteristics of patients with psychogenic nonepileptic seizures. *Epilepsia* 1999; 40(9): 1292–8.

Gaynor D, Cock H, Agrawal N. Psychological treatments for functional non-epileptic attacks: a systematic review. *Acta Neuropsychiatrica* 2009; 21(4): 158–68.

Krumholz A. Nonepileptic seizures: diagnosis and management. *Neurology* 1999; 53(5, Suppl 2); S76–S83.

Reuber M, House AO. Treating patients with psychogenic non-epileptic seizures. *Current Opinion in Neurology* 2002; 15: 207–11.

Useful websites

Functional and Dissociative Neurological Symptoms: a aptient's guide. www.neurosymptoms.org (accessed 28 March 2011).
NEAD Trust: http://www.neadtrust.co.uk/ (accessed 28 March 2011).

References

1. Aldenkamp AP, Mulder OG. Behavioural mechanisms involved in pseudo-epileptic seizures: a comparison between patients with epileptic seizures and patients with pseudo-epileptic seizures. *Seizure* 1997; 6: 275–82.

2. Martin RC, Gilliam FG, Kilgore M, Faught E, Kuzneicky,R. Improved health care resource utilisation following video-EEG-confirmed diagnosis of non-epileptic psychogenic seizures. *Seizure* 1998; 7: 385–90.
3. Szaflarski JP, Hughes C, Szaflarski M et al. Quality of life in psychogenic nonepileptic seizures. *Epilepsia* 2003; 44: 236–42.
4. Witgert ME, Wheless JW, Breier JI. Frequency of panic symptoms in psychogenic nonepileptic seizures. *Epilepsy and Behavior* 2005; 6: 174–8.
5. Benbadis SR, Hauser WA. An estimate of the prevalence of psychogenic nonepileptic seizures. *Seizure* 2000; 9: 280–1.
6. Sigurdardottir KR, and Olafsson E. Incidence of psychogenic seizures in adults: a population-based study in Iceland. *Epilepsia* 1998; 39(7): 749–52.
7. Frolov MV, Korinevskaya IV, Vorob'eva OV. Phenomenological assessment of psychogenic paroxysms using parameters of verbal activity. *Human Physiology* 2003; 20(1): 26–30.
8. Kato M. Epilepsy and pseudoseizures derived from their dissociation. *Psychiatria et Neurologia Japonica* 2006; 108(3): 251–9.
9. Kuloglu M, Atmaca M, Tezcan E, Gecici O, Bulut S. Sociodemographic and clinical characteristics of patients with conversion disorder in eastern Turkey. *Social Psychiatry and Psychiatric Epidemiology* 2003; 38: 88–93.
10. Silva W, Giagante B, Saizar R et al. Clinical features and prognosis of nonepileptic seizures in a developing county. *Epilepsia* 2001; 42(3): 398–401.
11. Yeh EA. Pseudoseizures in social and cultural context. *Transcultural Psychiatric Research Review* 1996; 33(1): 3–32.
12. Galimberti CA, Ratti MT, Murelli R, Marchioni E, Manni R, Tartara A. Patients with psychogenic nonepileptic seizures, alone or epilepsy-associated, share a psychological profile distinct from that of epilepsy patients. *Journal of Neurology* 2003; 250: 338–46.
13. Schwabe M, Howell SJ, Reuber M. Differential diagnosis of seizure disorders: A conversation analytic approach. *Social Sciences and Medicine* 2007; 65: 712–24.
14. Sen A, Scott K, Sisodiya SM. Stertorous breathing is a reliably identified sign that helps in the differentiation of epileptic from psychogenic non-epileptic convulsions: an audit. *Epilepsy Research* 2007; 77: 62–4.
15. American Psychiatric Association. *Diagnostic and Statistical Manual of Mental Disorders*, 4th edn, text revision). Washington, DC: American Psychiatric Association; 2000.
16. World Health Organization. *ICD-10. International Statistical Classification of Diseases and Related Heath Problems*, 10th revised edition). Geneva: World Health Organization; 1992.
17. Bowman ES, Markand ON. Psychodynamics and psychiatric diagnoses of pseudoseizure subjects. *American Journal of Psychiatry* 1996; 153: 57–63.
18. Mökleby K, Blomhoff S, Malt UF, Dalström A, Tauböll E, Gjerstad L. Psychiatric comorbidity and hostility in patients with psychogenic nonepileptic seizures compared with somatoform disorders and healthy controls. *Epilepsia* 2002; 43(2): 193–8.
19. Jawad SSM, Jamil N, Clarke EJ, Lewis A, Whitecross S, Richens A. Psychiatric morbidity and psychodynamics of patients with convulsive pseudoseizures. *Seizure* 1995; 4: 201–206.
20. Buchanan N, Snars J. Pseudoseizures (non-epileptic attack disorder): clinical management and outcome in 50 patients. *Seizure* 1993; 2:141–8.

21. Roy A, Barris M. Psychiatric concepts in psychogenic nonepileptic seizures. In: Rowan AJ, Gates JR, eds. *Non-epileptic seizures*. Boston: Butterworth-Heinemann, 1993: 143–151.
22. Prueter C, Schultz-Venrath U, Rimpau W. Dissociative and associated psychopathological symptoms in patients with epilepsy, pseudoseizures, and both seizure forms. *Epilepsia* 2002; 43(2): 188–92.
23. Bowman ES. Nonepileptic seizures: psychiatric framework, treatment, and outcome. *Neurology* 1999;53(5 Suppl 2): S84–S88.
24. Derry PA, McLachlan RS. The MMPI-2 as an adjunct to the diagnosis of pseudoseizures. *Seizure* 1996; 5: 35–40
25. Kalogjera-Sackellares D, Sackellares C. Personality profiles of patients with pseudoseizures. *Seizure* 1997; 6: 1–7.
26. Alper K, Devinsky O, Perrine K, Vazquez B, Luciano D. Psychiatric classification of nonconversion nonepileptic seizures. *Archives of Neurology* 1995; 52(2): 199–201.
27. Krumholz A. Nonepileptic seizures: diagnosis and management. *Neurology* 1999; 53(5 Suppl 2): S76–S83.
28. van Rijckevorsel K, Lennox W, Fouchet P, Indriets J-P, Sylin M. Epidemiologic survey of a population of patients with nonepileptic attack disorders (NEADS): a contribution to psychological diagnosis. *Epilepsia* 1998; 39(s6): 181.
29. Wood BL, Haque S, Weinstock A, Miller BD. Pediatric stress-related seizures: conceptualization, evaluation, and treatment of nonepileptic seizures in children and adolescents. *Current Opinion in Pediatrics* 2004; 16: 523–531.
30. Teicher MH, Andersen SL, Polcari A, Anderson CM, Navalta CP. Developmental neurobiology of childhood stress and trauma. *Psychiatric Clinics of North America* 2002; 25(2): 397–426.
31. Bowman ES. Etiology and clinical course of pseudoseizures: relationship to trauma, depression, and dissociation. *Psychosomatics* 1993; 34(4): 333–42.
32. Moore PM, Baker GA. Nonepileptic attack disorder: a psychological perspective. *Seizure* 1997; 6: 429–34.
33. Salmon P, Al-Marzooqi SM, Baker G, Reilly J. Childhood family dysfunction and associated abuse in patients with nonepileptic seizures: toward a causal model. *Psychosomatic Medicine* 2003; 65: 695–700.
34. Gaynor D, Cock H, Agrawal N. Psychological treatments for functional nonepileptic attacks: a systematic review. *Acta Neuropsychiatrica* 2009; 21(4): 158–68.
35. Shen W, Bowman ES, Markand ON. Presenting the diagnosis of pseudoseizure. *Neurology* 1990; 40: 756–9.
36. Ataoglu A, Ozectin A, Icmeli C, Ozbulut O. Paradoxical therapy in conversion reaction. *Journal of Korean Medical Science* 2003; 18: 581–4.
37. Brown RJ, Trimble MR. Dissociative psychopathology, non-epileptic seizures, and neurology. *Journal of Neurology, Neurosurgery and Psychiatry* 2000; 69: 285–91.
38. Goldstein LH, Deale AC, Mitchell-O'Malley SJ, Toone BK, Mellers JDC. An evaluation of cognitive behavioral therapy as a treatment for dissociative seizures. *Cognitive Behavioral Neurology* 2004; 17(1): 41–9.
39. LaFrance WC Jr, Miller IW, Ryan CE et al. Cognitive behavioral therapy for psychogenic nonepileptic seizures. *Epilepsy and Behavior* 2009; 14: 591–6.

146   *Danielle Gaynor and Niruj Agrawal*

40. Chabolla DR, Krahn LE, So EL, Rummans TA. Psychogenic nonepileptic seizures. *Mayo Clinic Proceedings* 1996; 71(5): 493–500.
41. Ettinger AB, Dhoon A, Weisbrot DM, Devinsky O. Predictive factors for outcome of nonepileptic seizures after diagnosis. *Journal of Neuropsychiatry and Clinical Neuroscience* 1999; 11(4): 458–63.
42. LaFrance WC, Barry JJ. Update on treatments of psychological nonepileptic seizures. *Epilepsy and Behaviour* 2005; 7: 364–74.
43. Brown RJ. Psychological mechanisms of medically unexplained symptoms: an integrative conceptual model. *Psychological Bulletin* 2004; 130(5): 793–812.
44. Ramani V, Gumnit RJ. Management of hysterical seizures in epileptic patients. *Archives of Neurology* 1982; 39(2): 78–81.
45. Drake ME, Pakalnis A, Phillips BB. Neuropsychological and psychiatric correlates of intractable pseudoseizures. *Seizure* 1992; 1: 11–13.
46. LaFrance WC, Devinsky O. Treatment of nonepileptic seizures. *Epilepsy and Behavior* 2002; 3: S19–S23.
47. Stonnington CM, Barry JJ, Fisher RS. Conversion disorder. *American Journal of Psychiatry* 2006; 163(9): 1510–17.
48. Alsaadi TM, Marquez AV. Psychogenic nonepileptic seizures. *American Family Physician* 2005; 72(5): 849–56.
49. Silver FW. Management of conversion disorder. *American Journal of Physical Medicine and Rehabilitation* 1996; 75(2): 134–40.
50. Rusch MD, Morris GL, Allen L, Lathrop L. Psychological treatment of nonepileptic events. *Epilepsy and Behaviour* 2001; 2: 277–83.
51. Alper K, Devinsky O, Perrine K, Vazquez B, Luciano D. Nonepileptic seizures and childhood sexual and physical abuse. *Neurology* 1993; 43: 1950–3.
52. Reuber M, House AO. Treating patients with psychogenic non-epileptic seizures. *Current Opinion in Neurology* 2002; 15: 207–211.
53. Wood BL, McDaniel S, Burchfiel K, Erba G. Factors distinguishing families of patients with psychogenic seizures from families with epilepsy. *Epilepsia* 1998; 39(4): 432–7.
54. Buchanan N, Snars J. Pseudoseizures (non-epileptic attack disorder): clinical management and outcome in 50 patients. *Seizure* 1993; 2: 141–8.
55. Turgay A. Treatment outcome for children and adolescents with conversion disorder. *Canadian Journal of Psychiatry* 1990; 35: 585–9.
56. Moore PM, Baker GA, McDade G, Chadwick D, Brown S. Epilepsy, pseudoseizures and perceived family characteristics: a controlled study. *Epilepsy Research* 1994; 18(1): 75–83.
57. Owczarek K. Somatisation indexes as differential factors in psychogenic pseudoepileptic and epileptic seizures. *Seizure* 2003; 12: 178–81.
58. Taylor S, Garralda E. The management of somatoform disorder in childhood. *Current Opinion in Psychiatry* 2003; 16: 227–31.
59. Kozlowska K, Nunn KP, Rose D, Morris A, Ouvrier RA, Varghese J. Conversion disorder in Australian pediatric practice. *Journal of the American Academy of Child and Adolescent Psychiatry* 2007; 46(1): 68–75.
60. Goldstein LH, Drew C, Mellers J, Mitchell-O'Malley S, Oakley, D. Dissociation, hypnotizability, coping styles, and health locus of control: characteristics of pseudoseizure patients. *Seizure* 2000; 9: 314–22.

61. Kuyk J, Spinhoven P, van Dyck R. Hypnotic recall: a positive criterion in the differential diagnosis between epileptic and pseudoepileptic seizures. *Epilepsia* 1999; 40(4): 485–91.
62. Black DN, Seritan AL, Taber KH, Hurley RA. Conversion hysteria: lessons from functional neuroimaging. *Journal of Neuropsychiatry and Clinical Neuroscience* 2004; 16: 245–51.
63. Walczak TS, Papacostas S, Williams DT, Scheuer ML, Lebowitz N, Notarfrancsco A. Outcome after diagnosis of psychogenic nonepileptic seizures. *Epilepsia* 1995; 36(11): 1131–7.
64. Myers L, Zaroff C. The successful treatment of psychogenic nonepileptic seizure using a disorder-specific treatment modality. *Brief Treatment and Crisis Intervention* 2004; 4(4): 343–52.
65. Bhatia MS, Sapra S. Pseudoseizures in children: a profile of 50 cases. *Clinical Pediatrics* 2005; 44(7): 617–21.
66. Wittenberg D, Michaels J, Ford C, Bullock K, Barry JJ. Group psychotherapy for patients with non-epileptic seizures: a pilot study. *Epilepsia* 2004; 45(s7): 57–8.
67. Wolanczyk T, Brynska A. Psychogenic seizures in obsessive-compulsive disorder with poor insight: a case report. *Pediatric Neurology* 1998; 18(1): 85–6.
68. Betts T, Boden S. Diagnosis, management and prognosis of a group of 128 patients with non-epileptic attack disorder. Part I. *Seizure* 1992; 1: 19–26.
69. McDade G, Brown SW. Non-epileptic seizures: management and predictive factors of outcome. *Seizure* 1992; 1: 7–10.
70. LaFrance WC, Devinsky O. Treatment of nonepileptic seizures: historical perspectives and future directions. *Epilepsia* 2004; 45(s2): 15–21.
71. Farias ST, Thieman C, Alsaadi TM. Psychogenic nonepileptic seizures: acute change in event frequency after presentation of the diagnosis. *Epilepsy and Behaviour* 2003; 4: 424–9.
72. Ettinger AB, Devinsky O, Weisbrot DM, Ramakrishna RK, Goyal A. A comprehensive profile of clinical, psychiatric, and psychosocial characteristics of patients with psychogenic nonepileptic seizures. *Epilepsia* 1999; 40(9): 1292–8.
73. Krumholz A, Neidermeyer E. Psychogenic seizures: a clinical study with follow-up data. *Neurology* 1983; 33(4): 498–502.
74. Jongsma MJ, Mommers JM, Renier WO, Meinardi H. Follow-up of psychogenic, non-epileptic seizures: a pilot study – experience in a Dutch special centre for epilepsy. *Seizure* 1999; 8: 146–8.
75. Reuber M, Pukrop R, Bauer J, Helmstaedter C, Tessendorf N, Elger CE. Outcome in psychogenic nonepileptic seizures: 1 to 10 year follow-up in 164 patients. *Annals of Neurology* 2003; 53: 305–311.

8
Gilles de la Tourette Syndrome

Jeremy S. Stern and Mary M. Robertson

Tourette syndrome (TS) has a distinctive history – originally described in a noble woman, the Marquise de Dampierre in 1825 by Itard, with a series of several more patients presented by Gilles de la Tourette in 1885 from the Salpêtrière hospital, probably under the wing of Charcot. The Marquise was included in this second series, she lived to an old age and was socially very confined by her involuntary swearing. The condition was considered a very rare and bizarre curiosity for many years, with few case reports and what we would consider today to be an inappropriate and unfortunate psychodynamic interpretation and consequent treatment. In the 1970s there was a resurgence of interest in New York. By the 1980s the generally accepted prevalence was 1 in 2000 but, more recently, as described below, this has been found to be a serious underestimate.

There has been a consequent mushrooming in the literature. A PubMed search in September 2007 using the word 'Tourette' identified no fewer than 2876 publications. In a wide review such as this, it is necessary to limit the number of references cited; therefore, for the details of much important data, the reader is necessarily directed to other reviews. The original publications included are necessarily arbitrary but hopefully give a representative picture of progress over the last 20 years, with particular emphasis on recent advances in understanding and management.

Clinical phenomenology and diagnosis

The current internationally accepted diagnostic criteria for TS include multiple motor tics and one or more vocal (phonic) tics, which last longer than a year (*Diagnostic and Statistical Manual of Mental Diseases,*

4th edition text revision [DSM-IV-TR][1] Box 8.1). Tics are involuntary, usually brief, twitch-like movements that nevertheless can also usually be suppressed for short periods of time. Suppression tends to be associated with a sense of rising inner tension and is followed by a rebound in severity. Tics are rather situational, for instance worse in a stressful situation and better when the individual is mentally absorbed, such as while playing music or sport, or driving. They wax and wane over short and longer time periods, with new tics appearing and old ones remitting.

The age at onset of TS ranges from 2 to 21 years, with a mean of 5–7 years commonly reported. In an important early series known as the International Registry (IR), Abuzzahab and Anderson reported that 90% of symptoms began between the ages of 3 and 16 years.[2] The onset of vocal tics is usually later, often at around 11 years. Tics can be simple or complex, and premonitory sensations, which may be localised or generalised, are common. The most common motor tics are blinking, head nodding and facial grimacing, while sniffing, throat clearing and coughing are the most common vocal tics. Other features include echolalia (copying what other people say), echopraxia (copying what other people do, for example, facial expressions) and palilalia (repeating the last word or phrase that oneself has uttered). In the IR, the most common motor tics involved the face (92%), followed by the arms (78%), and vocal tics included inarticulate utterances (65%) and echolalia (23%).[2]

Coprolalia is the inappropriate use of obscenities, which the patient often attempts to disguise. It is usually distressing and has a different quality to excessive swearing in a social sense, often being completely outside normal grammatical context. It was once thought to be necessary for the diagnosis of TS, but in fact only occurs in approximately

---

Box 8.1   DSM-IV-TR diagnostic criteria for Tourette syndrome[1]

A. Both multiple motor and one or more vocal tics have been present at some time during the illness, although not necessarily concurrently. (A *tic* is a sudden, rapid, recurrent, non-rhythmic, stereotyped motor movement or vocalisation.)
B. The tics occur many times a day (usually in bouts) nearly every day or intermittently throughout a period of more than 1 year, and during this period there is never a tic-free period of more than 3 consecutive months.
C. The onset is before the age of 18 years.
D. The disturbance is not due to the direct physiological effects of a substance (e.g. stimulants) or a general medical condition (e.g. Huntington's disease or postviral encephalitis).

10–15% of TS patients overall, and 30% of specialist TS clinic patients. Coprolalia usually starts at the age of around 15 years.[3] In the IR, coprolalia was present in 58% but at that time many clinicians mistakenly understood that coprolalia was necessary to make the diagnosis, and thus a higher incidence of the symptom would be expected. There have been suggestions that the content of coprolalia may be modified by cultural and psychosocial factors.[3]

Recent evidence from studies employing hierarchical cluster analyses and principal-component factor analyses on consecutive cohorts of patients[4] and large families multiply affected with TS, have challenged the notion that TS is a unitary condition by the demonstration of several heritable factors amongst groups of different symptoms and tic types. This would suggest separate distinguishable phenotypes. These findings have major implications for genetics studies compounding the difficulty in phenotype definition, more so as the condition has major comorbidities (see below), which can be present in family members in the absence of tics.

Self-injurious behaviours (SIBs) have been shown to be significantly associated with obsessionality as well as impulsivity and poor impulse control. Some SIBs appear not to be related to the severity of TS, as even in mildly affected family members in a large pedigree, SIB significantly differentiates between cases of TS and non-cases. Eye SIB appears to be common.[3] The behaviours appear to be different from the self-mutilation and deliberate self-harm encountered in other psychiatric disorders, which include self-cutting (in the setting of personality disorders [PDs]), overdosing in both depression or PDs, and lip biting in Lesch–Nyhan syndrome.

In DSM-IV, both impairment and distress were included in the diagnostic criteria, but these have been omitted from DSM-IV-TR.[1] The highest age at onset has differed in the various DSM criteria, but all have dictated that TS must begin under the age of 21 years. Adult-onset tic disorders are not well documented and are atypical.

DSM definitions of other tic disorders include transient tic disorder,[1] which is more common in children than TS, and by definition lasts less than a year, and chronic motor or vocal tic disorder (CMT),[1] in which motor and vocal tics are not combined. The vast majority of the literature centres on TS.

Epidemiology

The changing conception of the frequency of TS is perhaps epitomised by the IR only 21 years ago,[2] in which a mere 430 TS cases were documented worldwide. By 2000 the International TIC Consortium had documented 3500 cases.[5] Not all clinicians seeing cases worldwide belong to the consortium, and using most recent epidemiological data it is clear that the global prevalence is far higher. In any case, many cases of TS, particularly mild cases, are unknown to medical services and there are many more than have been documented. In our opinion, it is unlikely that TS has become more common, but more likely that recognition has improved.

TS occurs worldwide,[2,5] but few cases have been documented in sub-Saharan black Africans (Robertson, 1996; unpublished data). In almost all studies, there is a male predominance of 3–4:1 or 70%.[2]

In recent epidemiological studies, a prevalence of between 0.46% and 1.85% for children between the ages of 5 and 18 years has been suggested. The prevalence of TS in special educational populations and people with autistic spectrum disorder (ASD) is substantially higher.[3]

In conclusion, TS is no longer considered rare and in fact should be thought of as not uncommon, but, in general, milder cases are probably unknown to medical services. The clinical phenomenology is similar worldwide, emphasising the biological underpinnings of the disorder.

Psychopathology

Few individuals with TS in clinics have no other problems. The International TIC Consortium of 3500 TS clinic patients demonstrated that 88% had comorbidity.[5] The most common was ADHD (attention deficit hyperactivity disorder), followed by obsessive-compulsive behaviour (OCB) and OCD. Anger-control problems, sleep difficulties, coprolalia and SIB only reached high levels in individuals with comorbidity. In a more recent Swedish epidemiological study, the prevalence of TS was 0.6% of 4500 children aged between 7 and 15 years. Notably, only 8% of the TS patients identified in this community setting had no other diagnosis, while as many as 36% had three or more other diagnoses.[6] Thus, in both community and clinic settings, 88–92% of TS patients have other identifiable psychiatric diagnoses. A large Israeli study of young military recruits did show that comorbidities can occur in the context of mild undiagnosed TS, where the tics effectively act as a marker for the more serious impairments.[3]

Individuals with TS have increased anxiety, hostility and personality disorders.[3] Several have documented that although the OCB encountered in TS is integral to TS, it is significantly different from the behaviours encountered in 'pure' or 'primary' OCD.[3] The classic OCB in TS is characterised by 'evening up' (a concern with symmetry), getting things 'just right', forced touching of self and others and arithmomania (an obsession with numbers and counting), whilst in pure OCD the obsessions and compulsions are often to do with dirt, germs and contamination. Many of the TS patients with OCB do not find their symptoms distressing or bothersome and do not require treatment. In the Abuzzahab and Anderson IR, OCD was the most common comorbidity.[2] There is universal consensus that OCB/OCD and TS are genetically related in TS families.

The reasons for the high comorbidity between ADHD and TS are unclear, but the comorbidity does not necessarily point to one genetic cause, with only some cases appearing genetically related. A recent case control study of family histories of TS, ADHD and comorbidity concluded that the two conditions are not alternate phenotypes of one genotype but the two conditions do confer an increased risk of comorbidity, indicating some biological overlap.[7] The ADHD symptoms are often the ones that lead to social impairment. Sleep is also often disturbed in individuals with TS and particularly so if they also have ADHD.

Depression is common, with a lifetime risk of 10%, and prevalence of between 1.8% and 8.9%: depression or depressive symptoms occur in 13–76% of TS patients attending specialist clinics.[8] In a review of 13 controlled studies including 741 patients with TS, the TS patients were significantly more depressed than controls in all but one instance. In community and epidemiological studies, depression in TS individuals was less evident, occurring in two out of five investigations. Clinical correlates of the depression in people with TS included tic severity and duration, the presence of echo- and copro- phenomena, premonitory sensations, sleep disturbances, OCBs, SIB, aggression, conduct disorder (CD) in childhood, and possibly ADHD. The depression in people with TS was demonstrated to result in a lower quality of life (QOL), and may lead to hospitalisation and suicide.[8] The aetiology of depression appears to be multifactorial.

Although there have been reports of an association between bipolar affective disorder (BAD) and TS, there is little evidence of a wide association but BAD and TS may be related in some individuals.[8]

Dyslexia and dyspraxia are often said to be associated with TS, but few studies can confirm this anecdotal suggestion.[3] Nevertheless, patients are troubled by the symptoms and it possibly adds to generalised difficulties with education in some cases.

Inappropriate explosive outbursts of 'rage' are common in TS patients, although relatively few documentations of this exist. In general, there is a slight provocation, followed by a major outburst of 'rage', often followed by remorse. Clinically this is often one of the most difficult symptoms for the patient and the family, and to manage or treat.

The relationship between pervasive developmental disorders like autism and Asperger's syndrome and TS is complex, due to a clinical overlap in some respects, but TS can also emerge as a comorbidity. In a prevalence investigation, 447 pupils from nine schools for children and adolescents with autism were screened for the presence of motor and vocal tics. Results showed a diagnosis of definite TS in 19 children, giving a prevalence rate of 4.3%. A further 10 children were diagnosed with probable TS (2.2%). It was concluded that the combined rate of 6.5% TS in autism exceeded that expected by chance. The severity of autism had no bearing on the comorbidity and in the majority (>70%) of TS cases there was a positive family history of TS, tics or OCB/OCD.[9]

In conclusion, comorbid disorders of TS are complex and probably heterogeneous, and the precise relationships between TS and its associated psychopathologies are unclear in many instances.

Quality of life and family life

The only study formally investigating the QOL in over 100 people with TS used standardised schedules and demonstrated that patients with TS showed significantly worse QOL than a general population sample. The TS patients had better QOL than patients with intractable epilepsy, as measured by the standardised and accepted Quality of Life Assessment Schedule (QOLAS). Factors influencing QOL domains in TS patients were employment status, tic severity, OCB, anxiety and depression.[10]

Parents of children with TS have been examined for psychopathology in order to investigate the mental health and caregiver burden. In a cross-sectional cohort survey comparing the parents of children with TS to a control group from a paediatric asthma hospital outpatient clinic over a 6-month period, using the General Health Questionnaire (GHQ-28) and caregiver burden (Child and Adolescent Impact Assessment) scores, 76.9% of the parents of children with TS achieved caseness on the GHQ-28, compared with 34.6% of the parents of children with asthma; this effect remained significant after controlling for demographic variables. Parents of children with TS also experienced greater caregiver burden, and this burden was significantly correlated with GHQ caseness. It was concluded that parents of children with TS are at risk of psychiatric morbidity, and an intervention targeting caregiver burden was suggested to help reduce this.[11] These studies indicate that these aspects of the disorder (i.e. the consequences of TS on the patient and the family) are important. They are relatively under-researched and further work is suggested.

Neurobiology

Clinical investigations including structural neuroimaging, electroencephalography (EEG), CSF examination, etc are generally unremarkable. The fact that neuroleptics are an effective treatment has always lent a suspicion that dopamine transmission and basal ganglia dysfunction are central factors, although therapeutic effect alone is insufficient to prove this. Little postmortem tissue has been examined and studies are in single or very small numbers of brains. Recent studies have shown indications of a prefrontal and frontal dopaminergic abnormality and an increase in pallidal parvalbumin-positive cells (inhibitory interneurones), suggesting defective gamma amino butyric acid (GABA)ergic embryonic migration.[12]

Neuroimaging has been heavily exploited to further probe the locus of the pathology. The techniques have included volumetric magnetic resonance imaging (MRI) of series of patients, functional imaging using measurement of regional cerebral blood flow with positron emission tomography (PET), single photon emission computed tomography (SPECT) and functional MRI (fMRI), and lastly neurochemical imaging using PET and SPECT. Functional imaging of patients with TS can have varied interpretation according to the protocol used, as the measurement may reflect the state of ticcing or alternatively tic suppression, effects of neuroleptics in non drug-naïve subjects, or, what would be most interesting, the actual trait of having TS. Earlier studies were less sophisticated in this regard. Unsurprisingly, altered activity in striato-thalamo-cortical circuitry has been variably identified,[13] but the ultimate interpretation of what this means remains elusive in the authors' opinion. Neurochemical studies probing the contribution of perturbed dopamine systems have often been negative, but positive in some paradigms, and overall are thought to indicate increased dopaminergic innervation especially in the ventral striatum.[13]

Volumetric studies have a history of conflicting results, in part perhaps due to heterogeneous populations including variation in ages of subjects between studies. For instance, the cross-sectional area of parts of the corpus callosum has been found to be both increased and decreased in separate studies. There may be a trend towards the loss of normal asymmetry of volume of the deep brain structures. Most recently, there is a new concept of relating volumetric imaging to clinical course. The anterior caudate may be smaller (by about 5%), with size being inversely correlated with severity at 8-year follow-up, but not at the time of the scan.[14] The frontal cortical area is larger in children with TS, with an inverse relationship to severity. In adults there is change in the other direction. It is hypothesised that the increase in volume in children is a plastic response enabling tic suppression (also with compensatory hippocampal hypertrophy) and that where this fails, the patient is more likely to have a severe disorder in adulthood. These data are allied to fMRI and neuropsychological contributions.[15]

Another line of recent argument relates to the possibility of aberrant neural oscillation in TS, potentially ameliorated by effective treatment. This area has been explored elsewhere in the literature on movement disorders, and is beyond the scope of this review.[16]

Aetiology

The cause of the brain dysfunction underlying TS is unknown, and the nature of that dysfunction is still only accessible through speculation based on the data and concepts already discussed. One thing that is certain however, is that the syndrome is familial, with a genetic component in most cases. Other influences hypothesised to confer vulnerability to TS or increases in symptom severity are immunological/para-infectious mechanisms, pre- and perinatal difficulties, hormonal effects and psychosocial stressors.

Genetics

Complex segregation analyses of family history data provided strong evidence that the mode of transmission was compatible with an autosomal dominant with reduced penetrance model, but subsequent studies suggested that the mechanism of inheritance may be more complex. It is clear that TS has a significant genetic basis and that some individuals with TS, CMT and/or OCD manifest variant expressions of the same genetic susceptibility factors. Chromosomal abnormalities are very rare. Several areas of interest have been identified on 11 separate chromosomes (2, 4, 5, 7, 8, 10, 11, 13, 17, 18, 19), dopamine receptor D_2 gene polymorphisms, and the *DRD4* and *MOA-A* genes during six genome scans, and in further independent publications of candidate gene polymorphism association studies. The strongest most recent association is with region 2p using sib-analysis.[17] To date only one gene, *SLITRK1*, on chromosome 13q31.1 has been identified as causal in a small number of individuals with TS, but does not appear to be generally applicable.[18]

With the benefit of these six genome scans and other studies, it is suggested that many areas of interest may confer an increased risk for developing TS. The genetics of TS has clearly proved complex and there is almost certainly genetic heterogeneity that may well be the mechanism for parts of the clinical heterogeneity. By definition, this may underlie the disappointing failure, so far, to identify major single genes for this seemingly autosomal dominant condition.

Neuroimmunology

In the last decade, the possibility of a para-infectious mechanism mediated by anti-basal ganglia antibodies (ABGA) raised by group A beta-haemolytic streptococcal (GABHS) throat infection has evolved, in analogy to Sydenham's chorea, which itself is associated with neuropsychiatric features. The starting point was a newly described entity, called paediatric autoimmune neuropsychiatric disorders associated with streptococcal infections (PANDAS).[19] Interestingly, in contrast to TS, Sydenham's chorea itself is more common in girls.

More recently, other centres have found laboratory evidence of GABHS infections or ABGA in some patients with TS who do not fulfil the criteria of PANDAS, i.e. of abrupt onset in temporal association with throat infections. The majority of eight controlled studies have supported a role of GABHS and basal ganglia autoimmunity in a subgroup of TS patients, whilst others have failed to confirm the findings, leaving the area highly controversial with respect to pathogenicity, as the laboratory findings could be epiphenomenal. One study has examined phenotypic features of ABGA-positive and -negative patients. Fifty-three children and 75 adults with TS were examined. Twelve children (23%) and 18 adults (25%) with TS were ABGA positive. Disease duration, tic phenomenology and severity, frequency of echo/pali/coprophenomena, SIB and aggressive behaviour and frequency of OCD comorbidity did not significantly differ between ABGA-positive and -negative patients, except for ability to suppress tics (higher in ABGA-positive patients). Comorbid diagnoses of ADHD, oppositional defiant disorder (ODD) and CD were significantly less frequent in ABGA-positive patients. On multivariate logistic regression analysis, only ADHD remained inversely correlated with ABGA; this is one of the few studies to examine phenotypic manifestations in the light of presumed aetiological factors.[21]

Other investigators have suggested the potential role of pre- and perinatal events in the pathogenesis of TS, which include a wide variety of factors such as severe nausea and/or vomiting during the first trimester, premature low birth weight and low Apgar scores. One controlled study has been published, which showed that TS individuals had significantly more prenatal risk factors than a matched control group,[21] and prenatal smoking has also been implicated.

Given the difference in incidence in males and females, sex hormones have been considered as an aetiological factor and treatment suggestion, but no conclusion is possible yet. Stressful psychosocial life events have been documented as being associated with subsequent worse severity of depression, with lesser effects on tics and obsessionality.

Management

An approach to the management of TS must cover the whole spectrum of severity and comorbidity. Current accepted strategies include psychological therapies and drug treatment.

Given the range of severity of the condition, it is common for no active management to be required beyond explanation of the diagnosis. Unfortunately, with our current knowledge of the genetic basis of TS, definitive genetic counselling is not possible. Individuals with TS can be advised that there is an approximately 50% chance of transmitting the genetic factors to each child but because of reduced penetrance the genetic factors confer only an approximately 50% chance of expression of TS, reducing the risk to around 25% with milder rather than severe symptoms more likely.

The treatment of tics is hampered by a central feature that is probably under-represented in the literature, the variability of response to drugs between patients. The biological cause of this is unknown but presumably points, in some way, to the heterogeneity of the condition. Other factors have a major impact on the possibility of gathering rigorous evidence to guide management: namely, the tendency of the severity of tics to be widely variable in different patients, and to vary over time in each patient. Furthermore, it is difficult to objectively measure clinical change. There are a few validated instruments that attempt this by using physician rating (including the use of clinical video) and self-report questionnaires or a combination of the two. It is important to acknowledge that there is also variability of perceived impact of tics or comorbidity of a given severity, so the patient or parent will also guide the need for active treatment, but this is yet another factor that can confound clinical trials.

There have been a number of double blind randomised trials, often with small numbers and for short periods of time, sometimes with questionable endpoints, exposing the results to the biases dictated by the factors listed above. There have been fewer than 20 drug or placebo crossover trials, including trials of drugs that are not in common use. There are very many open-label trials of variable quality and case reports of a surprising number of drugs. This form of demonstration of efficacy has a distinct liability to overestimate the effectiveness of drugs and probably should be regarded as no more than a pilot study in most cases. This is not to say that clinical experience where clinicians have had the opportunity to treat many individuals has not been useful in identifying therapeutic candidates and developing know-how, but overall one must conclude that TS is an area that is not notable for evidence-based medicine.

It is not possible to comprehensively cite the literature here, nor would it be helpful to list every drug that has been proposed. Instead, some selected controlled trials will be mentioned, along with the authors' personal view of the field (Box 8.2).[3]

Box 8.2   Management of Tourette syndrome

Non-pharmacological
- e.g. habit-reversal training

Pharmacological
- Tics:
  - *neuroleptics*: haloperidol, sulpiride, pimozide, tiapride
  - *atypical agents*: risperidone, olanzapine, quetiapine, aripiprazole
  - *other*: tetrabenazine, botulinum toxin injection
  - *non-neuroleptic*: clonidine
- OCD:
  - *SSRIs*: fluoxetine, citalopram, fluvoxamine, paroxetine
  - *tricyclic antidepressants*: clomipramine
- ADHD:
  - *simulants*: methylphenidate, pemoline, dextroamfetamine
  - *non-stimulants*: atomoxetine, Clonidine

NB all drugs are started at lowest doses and increased slowly.
SSRI = selective serotonin reuptake inhibitor.

Non-drug treatment: habit-reversal training

Tourette syndrome passed, over two decades ago, through its history of being thought of as a psychological or non-organic entity. During that history, some psychodynamic therapies were proposed that do not fit into the model of the disease today. However, psychological and cognitive-behavioural treatments (CBT) have been found useful. CBT is certainly a valuable component in the treatment of OCD, but a number of approaches to helping tics have also been established, the foremost one being habit-reversal training (HRT), which has the most backing in the literature, including six randomised controlled trials, the largest of which had 43 subjects.[22] The elements of the treatment are awareness training (e.g. of premonitory sensations), competing response training, relaxation training, motivational techniques and social support. Perhaps counterintuitively, there is evidence for lack of a rebound or relapse of tics following successful treatment. Behavioural management and parent training may be used for comorbid ADHD.

Neuroleptics

Haloperidol was the first drug to be used for TS. There is no doubt that neuroleptic medication can be helpful for tics, sometimes dramatically. As already outlined, responses are variable between patients, and sometimes within patients at different times. Adverse effects can be problematic, although extrapyramidal effects appear rare.[3] Weight gain and depression are problems with several of the agents and should be discussed before initiation. Most neuroleptics can induce hyperprolactinaemia, but optimal management of this as an isolated finding is unclear. The authors check a baseline prolactin but do not routinely monitor, unless there is some indication. Drowsiness is not uncommon and can lead to discontinuation. The general rule is to start at very low doses and increase slowly. TS often tends to respond to smaller doses than psychosis.

Haloperidol itself is now little used in the United Kingdom (UK), due to adverse effects, and indeed there are controlled trial data to demonstrate the superiority of pimozide with similar efficacy.[3] Pimozide can be associated with electrocardiographic QT prolongation and electrocardiographic (ECG) monitoring is necessary. Sulpiride has been widely used in the UK. Given the landscape of small and uncontrolled trials in the literature, seemingly each new atypical neuroleptic has been reported. Probably the best information is regarding risperidone, which is felt to be potentially effective for tics and may also have a place in managing behavioural disturbance but does have a notable tendency to induce weight gain and may possibly be diabetogenic. Blood glucose should be monitored in patients with an obvious increase in weight.

The newest agent to excite interest is aripiprazole, which has an interesting pharmacology, acting predominantly as a partial agonist at dopamine D_2 and serotonin 5-HT_{1A} receptors and an antagonist at serotonin 5-HT_{2A} receptors. So far there are only open-label studies but it is certainly an agent worthy of further study.[23]

Clonidine

Clonidine is useful for both tics and hyperactivity and traditionally more used in the United States of America (USA). It is an α_2-noradrenergic agonist. As always, it should be started slowly but also withdrawn slowly because of the risk of rebound hypertension. Baseline and regular ECG monitoring is advised. Whilst it is an agent of first choice for comorbid TS and ADHD, the authors have found its effectiveness for tics disappointing in clinical practice. There is a trial to confirm this,[3] but also a randomised comparison showing similar efficacy to risperidone.

Stimulants and non-stimulants for ADHD

The use of stimulants (e.g. methylphenidate) has been felt controversial because of the possibility of this class of drug inducing tics or making them worse. As a result, children with tics are often excluded from trials of stimulants. The controversy has been largely tempered through a reappraisal of the natural history of tics and ADHD and randomised trial data confirming the theoretical risks were, in practice, overplayed.[24] Methylphenidate is also available in sustained-release preparations, which can be very convenient. The non-stimulant atomoxetine (a selective noradrenaline reuptake inhibitor) has been shown to be effective in children with TS and comorbid ADHD, and was also shown not to exacerbate tics, in a placebo randomised study of 128 patients,[25] which is the largest treatment trial in TS. Treatment of ADHD is a very important component of improving school function, often surpassing the need to treat tics. Management of ADHD in adults is somewhat controversial.

Selective serotonin reuptake inhibitors

SSRIs are used for OCD, preferably in higher doses with CBT as an adjunct. They can also be prescribed for depression. They do not seem to be primarily effective for tics but their anxiolytic effects may be of secondary value in ameliorating them.

Other drug treatments

As alluded to above, many drugs have been presented in open-label or retrospective trials. Crossover studies supportive of what we would consider non-mainstream options include baclofen,[26] and pergolide.[3] There has been other interest in dopamine agonists. The mechanism is unclear but an action at presynaptic receptors at low doses, causing inhibition of dopamine release, may be a possibility. Of drugs that do not reach this level of evidence, it is worth mentioning tetrabenazine, which has a monoamine-depleting effect with postsynaptic blockade and may be a helpful option.[3] It can, however, induce depression.

Polypharmacy and licensing issues in children

In order to treat tics and comorbidities effectively, the drug classes discussed here are frequently combined, with caution. There is not much evidence examining this but clinical practice has not in general identified significant safety concerns. Particular vigilance for extrapyramidal effects should be exercised if tetrabenazine is combined with neuroleptics. Another indication for polypharmacy is to attain augmentation effects, for example neuroleptics with an SSRI for OCD, or nicotine skin patch with neuroleptics for tics.[3] Prescribing for children can cause particular difficulties due to national pharmaceutical regulatory licensing arrangements – in the UK many of the drugs that have been commonly used are not specifically licensed or labelled for children with TS. In general, the reasons for this are to do with the expense to industry of obtaining new product licences and do not necessarily reflect what is already known about safety and efficacy. To date, the pharmaceutical industry has not marketed drugs for TS. If this changes there will be mixed benefits and dangers. The examples and implications of current licensing quirks will vary from country to country and may involve problematic negotiations of 'shared care' with primary care physicians.

Botulinum toxin injections

Botulinum toxin injection causes irreversible presynaptic blockade of acetylcholine release at motor endplates, which recovers over the course of weeks. Repeated injections are well established for treating dystonic conditions like torticollis. In TS, individual tics can be treated in this way not only through muscular paralysis but also, it seems, through reduction in the premonitory urge to tic. The limited literature is mixed in the overall effectiveness of this – in some patients the beneficial effects can be wider than the treated tic.[27] A particular specialist indication is laryngeal injection for intrusive vocal tics.[28]

Neurosurgery

A number of poorly documented neurosurgical approaches have been used over many years.[29] Apart from supposed treatments for tics, these have also included approaches for severe self-injurious OCD, for instance anterior cingulotomy/limbic leucotomy. However, in the current era of basal ganglia deep brain stimulation (DBS) for Parkinson's disease and certain dystonias, there is an ongoing explosion in interest in DBS for TS. The scientific problems are formidable – unlike Parkinson's disease there is no accepted experimental/anatomical model of the condition to allow a rational selection of the best surgical target, and all the provisos regarding the difficulty of controlled trials apply. One special form of control in this situation will be to insert DBS with the stimulation turned off for periods of time. There are already several case reports of successful implantation with dramatic results, and a case series of 18 patients.[30]

Prognosis

Several studies in the last two decades have suggested that the prognosis is better than once thought, with worst severity at 10–12 years and the majority of symptoms disappearing in half of the patients by the age of 18 years.[31] A more recent follow-up study of children after 7.6 years reported 85% had a reduction in tics during adolescence.[14] Only increased tic severity in childhood was associated with increased tic severity at follow-up. The average at worst tic severity was 10.6 years. However, worst-ever OCD symptoms occurred approximately 2 years later than worst tic severity. Increased childhood IQ was associated with increased OCD severity at follow-up. A community study also found that a younger age at onset is associated with more severe TS.[6] In the face of improving tics, the psychopathology, such as OCD, may persist severely until later and may also increase. There have been suggestions that OCD and depression in the setting of TS are related, and thus the TS patient may also be prone to depressive symptoms or depression later on in life, despite the fact that the tics may have lessened. No studies have explored this to date.

Conclusions

The literature on TS has expanded in concert with recognition that it is a relatively common condition, particularly in children, with many people improving in adolescence. While the genetics and neurobiology have yet to be solved, the body of current accumulated knowledge demands that patients with a problem severe enough to bring it to medical attention must be assessed to allow diagnosis and optimal management of the tics and other features. Adults with a severe disorder are a subgroup on their own but for the majority of patients the goal is to allow them to participate as far as possible in education and social development when young, so that when they reach an age where their tics decline they are in a position to fully engage in society and enjoy the best possible quality of life. Foreseeable developments are likely to centre on the role of neurosurgery in severe adult cases, further genetic discovery, continuing research using neuroimaging and resolution of the issue of ABGA/autoimmunity as a pathogenic factor.

Key learning points

Tourette syndrome is far more common than formerly believed and affects about 1% of schoolchildren.

Tourette syndrome is a genetic condition but the genetic mechanism is still unknown. There is current controversy over group A beta-haemolytic streptococcal induced basal ganglia autoimmunity as another possible aetiological factor, and pre- and perinatal factors may also contribute.

The majority of cases have comorbidities, most commonly OCD and ADHD.

Treatment is symptom orientated.

Tics can be treated with habit-reversal training, neuroleptics and clonidine.

Key references

Alsobrook JP 2nd, Pauls DL. A factor analysis of tic symptoms in Gilles de la Tourette's syndrome. *American Journal of Psychiatry* 2002; 159(2): 291–6.

● Khalifa N, von Knorring AL. Tourette syndrome and other tic disorders in a total population of children: clinical assessment and background. *Acta Paediatrica* 2005; 94(11): 1608–14.

Robertson MM. Tourette syndrome, associated conditions and the complexities of treatment. *Brain* 2000 ; 123(3): 425–62.

Swedo SE, Leonard HL, Garvey M et al. Pediatric autoimmune neuropsychiatric disorders associated with streptococcal infections: clinical description of the first 50 cases. *American Journal of Psychiatry* 1998; 155(2): 264–71.

www.tsa.org.uk (accessed 29 March 2010).

References

1. American Psychiatric Association. *Diagnostic and Statistical Manual of Mental Disorders*, 4th edn, text revision. Washington DC: American Psychiatric Association; 2002.
2. Abuzzahab FS Sr, Anderson FO. Gilles de la Tourette syndrome: cross cultural analysis and treatment outcome. In: Abuzzahab FS Sr, Anderson FO, editors. *Gilles de la Tourette's Syndrome Volume 1: international registry*. St Paul: Mason Publishing Co; 1976, p. 71–9.
3. Robertson MM. Tourette syndrome, associated conditions and the complexities of treatment. *Brain* 2000; 123(3): 425–62.
4. Alsobrook JP 2nd, Pauls DL. A factor analysis of tic symptoms in Gilles de la Tourette's syndrome. *American Journal of Psychiatry* 2002; 159(2): 291–6.
5. Freeman RD, Fast DK, Burd L, Kerbeshian J, Robertson MM, Sandor P. An international perspective on Tourette syndrome: selected findings from 3500 individuals in 22 countries. *Developmental Medicine and Child Neurology* 2000; 42(7): 436–47.
6. Khalifa N, von Knorring AL. Tourette syndrome and other tic disorders in a total population of children: clinical assessment and background. *Acta Paediatrica* 2005; 94(11): 1608–14.
7. Stewart SE, Illmann C, Geller DA, Leckman JF, King R, Pauls DL. A controlled family study of attention-deficit/hyperactivity disorder and Tourette's disorder. *Journal of the American Academy of Child and Adolescent Psychiatry* 2006; 45(11): 1354–62.
8. Robertson MM. Mood disorders and Gilles de la Tourette's syndrome: an update on prevalence, etiology, comorbidity, clinical associations, and implications. *Journal of Psychosomatic Research* 2006; 61(3): 349–58.
9. Baron-Cohen S, Scahill VL, Izaguirre J, Hornsey H, Robertson MM. The prevalence of Gilles de la Tourette syndrome in children and adolescents with autism: a large scale study. *Psychological Medicine* 1999 ; 29(5): 1151–9.
10. Elstner K, Selai CE, Trimble MR, Robertson MM. Quality of Life (QOL) of patients with Gilles de la Tourette's syndrome. *Acta Psychiatrica Scandinavica* 2001; 103(1): 52–9.
11. Cooper C, Robertson MM, Livingston G. Psychological morbidity and caregiver burden in parents of children with Tourette's disorder and psychiatric comorbidity. *Journal of the American Academy of Child and Adolescent Psychiatry* 2003; 42(11): 1370–5.
12. Kalanithi PS, Zheng W, Kataoka Y et al. Altered parvalbumin-positive neuron distribution in basal ganglia of individuals with Tourette syndrome. *Proceedings of the National Academy of Sciences of the United States of America*. 2005; 102(37): 13307–12.
13. Frey KA, Albin RL. Neuroimaging of Tourette syndrome. *Journal of Child Neurology* 2006; 21(8): 672–7.
14. Bloch MH, Leckman JF, Zhu H, Peterson BS. Caudate volumes in childhood predict symptom severity in adults with Tourette syndrome. *Neurology* 2005; 65(8): 1253–8.
15. Peterson BS, Choi HM, Hao XJ et al. Morphology of the amygdala and hippocampus in children and adults with Tourette syndrome. *Archives of General Psychiatry* 2007; 64(11): 1281–91.

16. Leckman JF, Vaccarino FM, Kalanithi PS, Rothenberger A. Annotation: Tourette syndrome: a relentless drumbeat – driven by misguided brain oscillations. *Journal of Child Psychology and Psychiatry, and Allied Disciplines* 2006; 47(6): 537–50.

17. Tourette Syndrome Association International Consortium for Genetics. Genome scan for Tourette disorder in affected-sibling-pair and multigenerational families. *American Journal of Human Genetics* 2007; 80(2): 265–72.

18. Deng H, Le WD, Xie WJ, Jankovic J. Examination of the *SLITRK1* gene in Caucasian patients with Tourette syndrome. *Acta Neurologica Scandinavica* 2006; 114(6): 400–402.

19. Swedo SE, Leonard HL, Garvey M et al. Pediatric autoimmune neuropsychiatric disorders associated with streptococcal infections: clinical description of the first 50 cases. *American Journal of Psychiatry* 1998; 155(2): 264–71.

20. Martino D, Defazio G, Church AJ et al. Antineuronal antibody status and phenotype analysis in Tourette's syndrome. *Movement Disorders* 2007; 22(10): 1424–9.

21. Burd L, Severud R, Klug MG, Kerbeshian J. Prenatal and perinatal risk factors for Tourette disorder. *Journal of Perinatal Medicine* 1999; 27(4): 295–302.

22. Himle MB, Woods DW, Piacentini JC, Walkup JT. Brief review of habit reversal training for Tourette syndrome. *Journal of Child Neurology* 2006; 21(8): 719–25.

23. Davies L, Stern JS, Agrawal N, Robertson MM. A case series of patients with Tourette's syndrome in the United Kingdom treated with aripiprazole. *Human Psychopharmacology* 2006; 21(7): 447–53.

24. Tourette's Syndrome Study Group. Treatment of ADHD in children with tics: a randomized controlled trial. *Neurology* 2002; 58(4): 527–36.

25. Allen AJ, Kurlan RM, Gilbert DL et al. Atomoxetine treatment in children and adolescents with ADHD and comorbid tic disorders. *Neurology* 2005; 65(12): 1941–9.

26. Singer HS, Wendlandt J, Krieger M, Giuliano J. Baclofen treatment in Tourette syndrome: a double-blind, placebo-controlled, crossover trial. *Neurology* 2001; 56(5): 599–604.

27. Marras C, Andrews D, Sime E, Lang AE. Botulinum toxin for simple motor tics: a randomized, double-blind, controlled clinical trial. *Neurology* 2001; 56(5): 605–10.

28. Porta M, Maggioni G, Ottaviani F, Schindler A. Treatment of phonic tics in patients with Tourette's syndrome using botulinum toxin type A. *Neurological Sciences* 2004; 24(6): 420–3.

29. Rauch SL, Baer L, Cosgrove GR, Jenike MA. Neurosurgical treatment of Tourette's syndrome: a critical review. *Comprehensive Psychiatry* 1995; 36(2): 141–56.

30. Servello D, Porta M, Sassi M, Brambilla A, Robertson MM. Deep brain stimulation in 18 patients with severe Gilles de la Tourette syndrome refractory to treatment: the surgery and stimulation. *Journal of Neurology Neurosurgery and Psychiatry* 2008; 79(2): 136–42.

31. Coffey BJ, Biederman J, Geller DA et al. The course of Tourette's disorder: a literature review. *Harvard Review of Psychiatry* 2000; 8(4): 192–8.

9
Depression in Physical Illness

Audrey Ng and Steven Reid

The link between depression and physical illness has been recognised since antiquity. Depression occurs frequently in physical illness but its diagnosis presents a challenge. It often presents with somatic complaints such as fatigue, insomnia and reduced appetite, which may be confused with signs of disease. There is also a common and misleading perception that is an understandable reaction to physical illness and does not require treatment.

Yet recognition is important, as depression in the medical setting has profound effects on patients, including impaired recovery, greater disability and a reduced quality of life. Patients with chronic medical illness and comorbid depression report a significantly greater symptom burden compared to those with medical illness alone, when controlling for severity of disease.[1] This may contribute to the increased medical investigations, hospital attendance and overall cost of health care in this patient group.[2] Furthermore, patients with comorbid physical illness and depression do respond to psychiatric treatments that may lead not only to alleviation in depressive symptoms but also an improvement in somatic symptoms and functional ability.

Epidemiology of depression in the physically ill

Studies have repeatedly demonstrated that patients with physical illness have increased rates of depression compared to community samples. Rates vary according to the setting and method of case finding, but diagnostic interview studies generally report a prevalence ranging from 10 to 15%, two to three times that in the general population. A similar proportion will have subclinical symptoms with a likelihood of developing future depression. A population-based study including over 100,000 subjects reported the prevalence of major depression in a number of long-term medical conditions (Figure 9.1).[3]

In contrast to previous studies this research found that young people have a particularly high prevalence of depression. Prevalence rates are also increased in specialist settings compared to primary care. This may in part be due to an association between depression and illness severity. However, patients with physical illness and depression are also more likely to worry about their symptoms and be dissatisfied with their treatment, and are less likely to adhere to treatment, thus increasing the likelihood that they will be referred to specialist services.

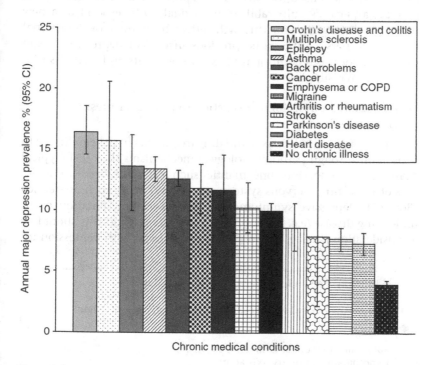

Figure 9.1 Prevalence of major depression in self-reported long-term medical conditions

Source: Adapted from Zigmond AS, Snaith RP. The hospital anxiety and depression scale. *Acta Psychiatrica Scandinavica* 1983; 67: 361–70.[4]

Note: COPD = chronic obstructive pulmonary disease.

The relationship between depression and physical illness

The link between physical illness and depressive symptoms can be conceptualised in a number of ways.

Depression as a psychological reaction to physical illness

Depression may be triggered in response to the diagnosis of a physical illness. An individual person's response will depend more on their perception of the illness than on the illness itself. Certain conditions are associated with a high degree of distress, notably conditions that are life-threatening, or disfiguring. Fear of the future, feelings of a loss of control, and a sense of failure are common responses to illness and do not inevitably lead to depression. As well as characteristics of the illness itself, of particular importance are risk factors that increase a person's vulnerability. Individuals will respond to a new diagnosis differently and this will reflect both their own personal resources – personality traits, previous history of depression – and external resources – additional stressful life events and lack of social and emotional support.

Depression as a physiological reaction to physical illness or its treatment

A number of physical illnesses and drug treatments have been linked to depression through pathophysiological mechanisms (Box 9.1). Typical examples are endocrine abnormalities such as hypothyroidism, disorders of the central nervous system, cancer, and drugs such as steroids (Box 9.2). Depressive symptoms may be the sole presentation of an underlying disease (e.g. carcinoma of the pancreas) and this should be a consideration particularly in people who present with depression for

---

Box 9.1   Depression and associated poor physical outcome

Depression is associated with negative physical outcomes through:

● *physiology*:
   – autonomic nervous system
   – hypothalamic pituitary axis activity
   – impairment in immune function

● *health-related behaviours*:
   – poor or unhealthy diet
   – smoking, alcohol, other substance misuse
   – reduced adherence to treatment.

the first time in later life. The role of prescription medicines in causing depression is frequently highlighted and merits consideration in assessment, although a direct cause–effect relationship has been definitively established for relatively few drugs.

Coincidental depression and physical illness

As both depression and physical illness are common in the general population, it is unsurprising that they frequently occur together. A thorough history will often find that the onset of depressive symptoms preceded the physical illness. Also, there is increasing evidence that major life events, such as bereavement, may precipitate physical as well as psychiatric illness.

Assessment

Screening

A systematic review found that routine use of screening questionnaires for depression had little influence on clinicians' behaviour and no

---

Box 9.2   Physical illnesses and drugs commonly associated with depression

Physical illnesses associated with depression

Intracranial

● Tumours
  Parkinson's disease
  Huntington's disease
  Cerebrovascular disease
  Encephalopathies (e.g. bovine spongiform encephalopathy [BSE])
● Head injury
  Multiple sclerosis

Extracranial

  Malignancy
  Endocrine disorders
  Infections (e.g. hepatitis B, infectious mononucleosis)

Drugs associated with depression

  Antihypertensives – reserpine, clonidine, propanolol, nifedipine
  Antiarrhythmics – digoxin, procainamide
  Anti-parkinsonian drugs – L-dopa, amantadine
  Cytotoxic agents – interferons, vincristine
  H_2-blockers – cimetidine
  Hormonal agents – corticosteroids, anabolic steroids, oral contraceptives
  Anticonvulsants – barbiturates, carbamazepine, vigabatrin
  Antiretroviral agents – nevirapine, efavirenz

impact on patient outcomes.[5] However, screening instruments can be of use for the detection of depression and a number of tools are available. The Hospital Anxiety and Depression Scale, developed specifically for use in the general hospital setting, omits questions about somatic symptoms that may be ambiguous indicators of depression in the physically ill.[4] The Beck Depression Inventory (BDI), frequently used in mental health settings, emphasises cognitive symptoms.[6] More recently, the Patient Health Questionnaire (PHQ) has been developed – commonly used in primary care it is a nine-item self-report measure that gives a tentative diagnosis of depression and indicates severity, which is particularly helpful in monitoring the response to treatment.[7]

The clinician should also be aware of covert indicators of a mood disorder in this group of patients, such as a failure to adjust to the illness, poorer physical functioning, a slower recovery than would be expected, and reduced social interaction or hostility towards staff.

Adjustment disorders

Distinguishing between a reactive state of distress and depression warranting specific treatment is often not straightforward. For many people faced with a physical illness, changes in mood are short-lived and resolve with an improvement in their physical symptoms. Adjustment disorders commonly follow the development of an acute illness or exacerbation of a chronic illness. A maladaptive reaction that, by definition, occurs within 3 months of an identifiable stressor, the characteristic symptoms include low mood, excessive anxiety, feelings of guilt and perhaps anger. These symptoms are self-limiting and should resolve within 6 months. Adjustment disorders may also manifest with reports of extreme helplessness, or denial of the existence of illness, but notably the symptoms are felt to be in excess of what would normally be expected and significantly interfere with social or occupational functioning. Attempting to define when psychological symptoms are in excess of what should be expected is often difficult and is particularly challenging in the context of a chronic illness with persisting disability. The treatment of adjustment disorders is primarily psychological and social, with a focus on non-specific support and information. However, when symptoms are persistent, severe or lead to significant disability, specific treatment for depression is indicated.

Diagnosis of depression

Five or more symptoms of depression that persist over a 2-week period are indicative of a depressive illness that warrants specific treatment

(Box 9.3). Of these, two symptoms are especially noteworthy: persistent, pervasive low mood and loss of interest or pleasure in usual activities (anhedonia). If the patient is depressed, the possibility that their symptoms may be directly due to a medical illness or its treatment should be considered (Box 9.2). Appropriate treatment of the underlying medical condition or a change of prescribed medication may be sufficient to alleviate the depression.

Somatic symptoms such as appetite loss and insomnia may be due to physical illness as well as depression, and thus may discriminate poorly between the two. Endicott suggested the substitutive approach to diagnosis (Box 9.3), replacing the somatic symptoms with additional cognitive or affective symptoms in medically ill patients. Although this method is effective, studies comparing diagnostic outcomes using both the regular and substituted criteria found that the rates of identification are similar, and there is no evidence that taking account of somatic complaints leads to over-diagnosis. In fact, depression comorbid with physical illness is more often missed for reasons such as misattribution of symptoms as a 'normal' response to illness, the stigma associated with a diagnosis of depression, unwillingness of patients to report symptoms, and unsuitability of the clinical setting for the discussion of emotional problems.

An important, but often neglected element of the assessment of depressed patients in the medical setting is the evaluation of suicidal

---

Box 9.3   Criteria for diagnosis of depression (based on Endicott J. Measurement of depression in patients with cancer. *Cancer* 1984; 53: 2243–9[8])

Persistent, pervasive depressed mood, decreased reactivity
Marked diminished interest or pleasure in activities
Fearful or depressed appearance
Diurnal variation in mood
Increased irritability, tearfulness
Social withdrawal or isolation, decreased talkativeness
Feelings of worthlessness, helplessness or hopelessness
Pessimism about the future, guilty feelings
Suicidal ideation or thoughts of self-harm

Biological symptoms that may be less discriminating

Weight loss or gain
Disturbed sleep
Fatigue, loss of energy
Poor concentration

thinking. Physical illness is an independent risk factor for suicide. In particular, patients with cancer, human immunodeficiency virus (HIV) and acquired immune deficiency syndrome (AIDS), chronic pain, and those undergoing renal dialysis are recognised to be especially vulnerable.

Specific illnesses associated with depression

Stroke

Both depression and anxiety occur commonly following a stroke. The risk of developing depression following stroke appears to be highest in the first few months of its occurrence.[9] Pooled data from prevalence studies of major depression post stroke indicate a frequency of 19% in the hospital setting and 14% in the community. When minor depression is taken into consideration, these figures rise to 35% and 32% respectively.[10] Post-stroke depression is a risk factor for poor functional and cognitive recovery as well as increased mortality.[11] The pathophysiology of post-stroke depression remains uncertain. Earlier studies reported an association with left anterior lesions, but this has been contradicted by a recent meta-analysis that found no such link.[12]

Antidepressant treatment following stroke needs to take into account both medical comorbidity and the potential for interaction with anticoagulants or cardiac drugs. Selective serotonin reuptake inhibitors (SSRIs) are generally well tolerated, and are indicated particularly in patients with significant heart disease. Citalopram is the SSRI least likely to interact with the anticoagulant warfarin. Tricyclic antidepressants are less likely to be used because of their potential for adverse anticholinergic and cardiac side effects, although there is no evidence for any difference in effectiveness. They also have a greater potential for lowering the seizure threshold. Some antidepressants, notably fluoxetine, citalopram and nortriptyline, have been used specifically for post-stroke depression to good effect. There is limited evidence that they may improve executive cognitive functioning independently of their effect on mood.[13]

Coronary heart disease

Numerous epidemiological studies have demonstrated that psychological factors and psychiatric illness affect the course and outcome of coronary heart disease. There is also significant evidence from prospective studies that major depressive disorder is an independent risk factor for the development of coronary heart disease, after controlling for lifestyle factors such as smoking and diet. In established coronary heart disease, the prevalence of major depression is 17–24%, and depression in these patients has an adverse effect on outcome, with increased risks of myocardial infarction. A similar prevalence of major depressive disorder has been found in patients following a myocardial infarction and an additional 20% will have minor depression or subthreshold depressive symptoms. Following an acute myocardial infarction, major depression has also been demonstrated to be a significant predictor of mortality in the first 6 months with a four-fold increase in risk, similar to the risk of a previous infarct.[14]

A number of mechanisms have been suggested as explanations for the effect of depression in coronary heart disease. In some patients depression may interfere with adherence to recommended management such as cardiac rehabilitation (and smoking cessation). Abnormalities of autonomic regulation mediated by depression may lead to alterations of resting heart-rate and heart-rate variability, which increase the risk of ventricular arrhythmias. A further possibility is that altered serotonin function in patients with depression makes them more vulnerable to serotonin-mediated platelet activation and subsequent vasoconstriction and thrombosis.

The safety and effectiveness of selective serotonin reuptake inhibitors in depressed patients with cardiovascular disease has now been established in a series of clinical trials: Sertraline Antidepressant Heart Attack Randomized Trial (SADHART), Enhancing Recovery in Coronary Heart Disease (ENRICHD), and Cardiac Randomized Evaluation of Antidepressant and Psychotherapy Efficacy (CREATE).[15–17] The problems associated with tricyclic antidepressants are well known: orthostatic hypotension, tachycardia, and, at high doses, cardiac arrhythmias. Most of the newer antidepressants such as venlafaxine, mirtazapine and duloxetine do not have the quinidine-like properties of the tricyclic antidepressants and are not associated with arrhythmias. However, they have not been extensively evaluated in patients with significant heart disease. Hypertension may occur with venlafaxine at higher doses, so patients receiving this drug should have periodic measurement of their blood pressure. In contrast to other physical illnesses, psychological interventions have an established history of use in cardiovascular disease through stress-management programmes. Cognitive-behavioural therapy (CBT) has also shown significant benefits in recent trials. What remains unclear, however, is whether effective treatment of depression in this population will have an effect on cardiovascular morbidity or mortality.

Parkinson's disease

Depression is a common neuropsychiatric complication of Parkinson's disease, with prevalence estimates as high as 40%. Studies have found that depression is one of the most important predictors of a poor quality of life in patients who suffer with Parkinson's disease, with evidence that it has as profound an effect as physical disability.[18] It is also associated with greater cognitive decline and progression of motor symptoms. Diagnosis is made difficult by the overlap of motor (bradykinesia, rigidity) and cognitive (impairment of concentration, apathy) symptoms with those of depression. During assessment, a focus on pervasive sadness, pessimistic thoughts and anhedonia may be helpful. Antiparkinsonian drugs may also have an adverse effect on the mental state. Levodopa and other dopamine-receptor agonists may cause hallucinations and depression.

There have been few trials of antidepressant treatment in patients with Parkinson's disease, so decisions about specific drugs should be made on a pragmatic basis. SSRIs are the preferred treatment option, given their favourable side-effect profile, although they may exacerbate tremor. They should be avoided in patients treated with selegiline (a monoamine oxidase B inhibitor) as there is a significant risk of serotonin syndrome and worsening extrapyramidal symptoms. Tricyclic antidepressants may be effective but caution should be exercised, as their anticholinergic properties can worsen cognitive problems, and alpha-blocking effects may worsen autonomic dysfunction.

Cancer

The assumption that 'patients with cancer manage well and few need help' is a myth. That depressive disorders are prevalent in patients diagnosed with a malignancy is unsurprising. Reported rates range from 20 to 50% according to cancer type and setting, but a survey of patients with a wide range of cancer types attending a regional oncology centre found an 8% prevalence of major depressive disorder using *Diagnostic and Statistical Manual of Mental Disorders*, 4th edition (DSM-IV) criteria.[19] Importantly, 85% of those cases identified were not receiving appropriate treatment for depression.

The outlook for many cancer patients is improving, with four out of every ten patients surviving the illness 5 years after diagnosis. Yet the diagnosis produces profound psychological stresses. Holland and colleagues described 'the six Ds', the universal fears experienced following a diagnosis of cancer: death, dependency on spouse or family, bodily disfigurement, disability, disruption of interpersonal relationships, and discomfort or pain.[20] Those who are at higher risk of depression are patients with poor physical condition, inadequate pain control, advanced stage of illness, and a previous history of depression. Carcinomas of the pancreas or lung, and head and neck malignancies are also associated with a markedly increased risk, due to pain, discomfort and disfigurement respectively. As anorexia, fatigue and weight loss are common to both cancer and depression, assessment should focus particularly on psychological symptoms. Perhaps more so than in other illness, patients with cancer are particularly likely to assume a responsibility to cope and are often reluctant to communicate symptoms of depression. Studies in breast and lung cancer have shown that both depression and a depressive 'coping style' are significantly associated with reduced survival. In contrast, there is no indication that a non-depressive coping style or 'fighting spirit' is beneficial.

Cognitive-behavioural and problem-solving therapies are the most commonly researched psychological treatments in comorbid depression and cancer. Moorey and Greer developed a cognitive-behavioural treatment specifically for cancer patients, which focuses on the personal meaning of the cancer for the individual and the patient's coping strategies, and some trials are encouraging, though there are studies that have not replicated this finding.[21] As it is important to minimise drug interactions, citalopram and sertraline would be a reasonable first choice to treat depressive symptoms in patients with cancer. Complementary therapies such as aromatherapy and reflexology have gained in popularity in recent years for the treatment of cancer in depressed patients but evidence supporting their use is scarce and the value of such therapies warrants further examination.

Diabetes

Diabetes mellitus is a heterogeneous metabolic disease in which hyperglycaemia is the central feature. It is a major public health problem with an increasing incidence, due to rising rates of obesity, an increasingly sedentary lifestyle, and an ageing population. Depressive symptoms are commonly described in association with diabetes and there is a substantial body of research showing that depression is associated with an increased risk of diabetic complications: retinopathy, neuropathy and renal impairment. What is less clear is whether depression increases the risk of complications through poor glycaemic control, or whether poorly managed diabetes and its complications lead to depressive disorders. There is also evidence from epidemiological studies suggesting that major depression is an independent risk factor for type 2 diabetes.

SSRIs are the preferred antidepressant treatment in diabetes as they are less likely to affect glucose metabolism. Caution should be exercised with fluoxetine, as it has been associated with an increased incidence of hypoglycaemia. Tricyclic antidepressants impair diabetic control as they may increase serum glucose. They also cause increased appetite and carbohydrate craving. Of the newer antidepressants, weight gain is often reported with mirtazapine. Tricyclics are often used for management of the painful neuropathies associated with diabetes. Randomised trials have shown their effectiveness while SSRIs show no difference from placebo. More recently, duloxetine has been licensed for the treatment of diabetic peripheral neuropathy.

HIV/AIDS

Rates of major depression in HIV infection vary from 5 to 35%, depending on the sampling criteria used and the stage of illness. Previously considered a terminal illness requiring palliative care, the advent of highly active antiretroviral therapy (HAART) has transformed the natural history of the disease. For many patients, at least in the developed world, living with HIV disease presents many of the challenges and impairments of physical and social functioning associated with other chronic illnesses.

A significant association has been found between HIV-related physical symptoms and the severity of depressive symptoms, but there is no evidence that depression has an impact on disease progression. The significantly increased suicide rate associated with HIV infection indicates the importance of a risk assessment in this group, taking account of factors such as depression, isolation, substance misuse and the stigma associated with HIV. The antiretroviral drugs used in HIV infection commonly cause fatigue and sleep disturbance. Nevirapine and efavirenz are both associated with psychiatric adverse effects, notably depressed mood and psychotic symptoms.

A meta-analysis of randomised controlled trials of antidepressant medication among HIV-positive individuals concluded that antidepressants were efficacious in treating depression, with studies using fluoxetine, paroxetine and imipramine showing good results.[22] In comparison with tricyclic antidepressants, SSRIs are more tolerable and have fewer adverse effects, which may improve adherence to treatment. Citalopram and sertraline in particular have a low potential for interaction with antiviral treatment, in contrast to many of the older antidepressants, notably monoamine oxidase inhibitors.

Although CBT has been shown to be effective for the treatment of depression and anxiety in the general population, there have been few trials of its use in HIV populations. One study found that interpersonal therapy was markedly effective compared to other psychological treatments, with the suggestion that a surfeit of HIV-related life events – multiple bereavements, role disputes and role transitions – made this treatment particularly suitable.[23] Distinct from psychological therapies, there is some evidence for the benefits of exercise, not only for physical health but also for psychological health. In a systematic review, aerobic exercise was linked to significant reductions in depressive symptoms, with potentially clinically important improvements in cardiopulmonary fitness for adults living with HIV or AIDS.[24]

Chronic pain

Disabling pain is a significant problem for many, with as many as one in five people in Europe affected by pain of longer than 6 months' duration. As well as the temporal criterion, chronic pain includes pains that have persisted for a month beyond the usual course for injury or acute illness, pain associated with a chronic pathological process, and pain that recurs episodically over months or years. For most complaints of chronic pain, however, there is no demonstrable pathology. Depression and chronic pain frequently co-occur, regardless of whether there is a clear organic basis for the pain. The prevalence of major depression in various groups of chronic pain patients varies from 8 to 50% and is dependent on the type and location of pain, and in particular the sample investigated and the method of assessment of depression. The causal pathway between chronic pain and depression is reciprocal: as well as pain being an established precursor of depression, depressed patients are more likely to complain of pain, seek medical help for the pain and have a lower perception of their ability to manage pain. Notably, there is strong evidence that chronic pain patients are at significantly increased risk for the presence of suicidal ideation and completed suicide.

Antidepressants have an important role in the management of depression associated with chronic pain. Tricyclic antidepressants have well-established analgesic properties in the absence of depression, as do some newer drugs, notably venlafaxine and duloxetine. In contrast, the SSRIs have no such effect. The multifactorial approach to chronic pain has led to the development of multidisciplinary pain clinics that combine the use of physical rehabilitation, medical management, cognitive-behavioural approaches and education. CBT has been found to be of particular benefit in addressing the mediating factors between depression and chronic pain. Coping styles such as catastrophising (the tendency to view pain and the individual's life situation as overwhelming), and idiosyncratic illness beliefs about pain – self-blame, helplessness – are related to depression, as are reduced levels of activity.

Management of depression in physical illness

Effective treatment of depression in patients with physical illness will improve not only psychological well-being but also their physical and social functioning and adherence to medical treatment. For patients with mild depression (four or fewer symptoms) and adjustment disorders, explanation, support and reassurance can reduce fear and uncertainty and may be all that is required as they are likely to recover with no specific intervention. For those with moderate or severe depression, management should include consideration of antidepressants as well as non-drug treatments.

Antidepressants

There is often a reluctance to use antidepressants in patients with physical illness, due to concerns about complicating treatment, adverse effects, or drug interactions. There is now an extensive body of evidence indicating that antidepressants in physical illness are effective and well tolerated.

A systematic review of 18 controlled studies concluded that treatment with tricyclic antidepressants or SSRIs led to significant improvements in depression associated with a range of physical illnesses, compared with placebo or no treatment.[25] It found that four patients (the number needed to treat) required treatment with antidepressants to produce one recovery from depression that would not have occurred had they been given a placebo.

There are a number of basic principles to consider when prescribing an antidepressant:

- discuss likely outcomes with the patient, e.g. gradual relief from depressive symptoms over several weeks
- antidepressants do not cause physical dependence
- prescribe a dose of antidepressant (after titration, if necessary) that is recognised as effective
- the antidepressant will need to be taken for at least 4–6 months to prevent any relapse of depression

● antidepressants must be taken regularly as prescribed and not just when the patient is feeling low.

In clinical practice, the choice of antidepressant will depend on the physical illness and drugs already prescribed, bearing in mind the potential for interactions. If patients are unable to accept oral administration of antidepressants, nasogastric or intravenous administration may be considered. Clomipramine, amitriptyline, citalopram and mirtazapine are all available for intravenous administration. SSRIs are usually the preferred choice of antidepressant due to their comparatively favourable side-effect profile. Newer antidepressants, such as reboxetine, should be used with caution, given that experience in patients with physical illness is limited. One of these, duloxetine, has also been licensed for treating pain, particularly in diabetic neuropathy as well as for urinary incontinence. Particular care is required in patients with renal, hepatic and cardiovascular disease, as outlined in Table 9.1.

St John's Wort (*Hypericum perforatum*) is a herbal preparation available over the counter for the treatment of depression. It has gained popularity in recent years and there is evidence that it is effective in treating mild to moderate depression. However, it is not advisable to recommend this drug as there is uncertainty about the appropriate dose, and available preparations vary markedly. Most importantly, it is a potent inducer of the hepatic cytochrome system and may interact with prescribed drugs causing serious adverse effects.

Electroconvulsive therapy

Recent years have seen the decline of the use of electroconvulsive therapy (ECT) although it remains an effective treatment for severe depression, particularly in the medical setting. ECT may be of particular benefit in instances where there has been profound weight loss or dehydration and a rapid definitive therapeutic response is required. In such cases, ECT may be a life-saving procedure. Although a safe treatment, there are some situations that require special justification for its use and due caution: raised intracranial pressure, recent myocardial infarction or intracerebral bleed, and other situations associated with a high anaesthetic risk.

Psychological treatment

CBT, interpersonal therapy, and problem-solving therapy have all shown effectiveness in the treatment of depression and are increasingly being used in medical settings. There has, however, been comparatively little study of their effectiveness in patients with physical illness.[26,27] The

Table 9.1   Use of antidepressants in selected medical disorders

	Selective serotonin reuptake inhibitors	Tricyclic antidepressants	Newer antidepressants[a]
Cardiovascular disease	SSRIs are generally considered safe and it is now advised that treatment should not be withheld post myocardial infarction (sertraline has no licensed restrictions) SSRIs have a mild anticoagulant effect	Should be avoided Increased risk of arrhythmias due to prolongation of QT and QRS intervals Reduce myocardial contractility Risk of postural hypotension	Venlafaxine should be avoided in patients with cardiovascular disease
Stroke	SSRIs considered safe Advise citalopram if patient taking warfarin	Nortriptyline has most supportive research evidence	Little data
Liver disease	Generally considered safe Use in renal disease with caution Avoid fluoxetine due to extensive hepatic metabolism and long half-life	Likelihood of increased sensitivity to adverse effects, particularly sedation, so should be used with caution	Dose reduction recommended
Renal disease	Generally considered safe to use with caution. Start with lower doses	Generally considered safe to use with monitoring for urinary retention, confusion, sedation and postural hypotension	Use with caution Venlafaxine should not be used in patients with electrolyte imbalance
Epilepsy	SSRIs should be used with caution though they have a low proconvulsive effect	Avoid in epilepsy as they reduce seizure threshold	Little data

potential benefits are clear: psychological treatments may be particularly useful where there are relative contraindications to antidepressants either because of physical illness or its treatment. Of these treatments, CBT has been most extensively investigated. There have been a number of randomised controlled trials demonstrating that this is an effective treatment for depression in patients with physical illness, particularly cancer.[28,29] These therapies also serve to support or improve coping strategies, an important aspect of treatment in physically ill patients. They are time consuming but in the longer term, compared with drug treatment, they may reduce the likelihood of relapse.

Conclusions

That depression is common in physical illness is now well recognised. The causes of depression in physical illness are complex: a combination of pathophysiological processes, overall burden of physical symptoms, a psychological reaction to a perceived loss, or external social stressors. What is clear, however, is that depressive disorders in patients with physical illness not only cause distress but also have an effect on overall health outcomes. Several longitudinal studies have shown that depression is more predictive of functional impairment over time than severity of physical illness. In addition, depression may increase the risk of mortality, as has been shown in the studies following myocardial infarction.

As is the case with the general population, depressed patients with comorbid physical illness often remain unrecognised and untreated. This is despite the availability of effective treatments for which there is growing evidence. Given the evidence for harms if left untreated, the recognition and treatment of depression in the physically ill should be a priority for clinicians.

Key learning points

- Depression is more common in people with physical illness than those without.
- Depression in physical illness should not simply be considered as an understandable reaction to circumstances, as it may have an adverse impact on prognosis.
- Depression in physical illness should be actively treated using antidepressant and/or psychological treatments.

● ECT is a safe and effective treatment for depression in physical illness and should be considered where there has been profound weight loss or dehydration and a rapid response is required.

Key references

Lloyd GG, Guthrie E, editors. *Handbook of Liaison Psychiatry*. New York: Cambridge University Press; 2007.

National Institute for Health and Clinical Excellence. *Depression in adults*. Clinical Guideline CG90. http://guidance.nice.org.uk/CG90/NICEGuidance/pdf/English

Taylor D, Paton C, Kerwin R. *The Maudsley Prescribing Guidelines*, 8th edn. Oxford: Taylor and Francis; 2005.

White CA. *Cognitive Behaviour Therapy for Chronic Medical Problems: a guide to assessment and treatment in practice*. Chichester: Wiley; 2001.

Patient Health Questionnaire (PHQ-9). http://www.depression-primarycare.org/clinicians/toolkits/materials/forms/phq9/ (accessed 30 March 2011).

References

1. Moussavi S, Chatterji S, Verdes E, Tandon A, Patel V, Ustun B. Depression, chronic diseases, and decrements in health: results from the World Health Surveys. *Lancet* 2007; 370: 851–8.
2. Creed F, Morgan R, Fiddler M, Guthrie E, House A. Depression and anxiety impair health-related quality of life and are associated with increased costs in general medical patients. *Psychosomatics* 2002; 43: 302–309.
3. Patten SB, Beck CA, Kassam A, Williams JVA, Barbui C, Metz LM. Long term medical conditions and major depression: strength of association for specific conditions in the general population. *Canadian Journal of Psychiatry* 2005; 50: 195–202.
4. Zigmond AS, Snaith RP. The hospital anxiety and depression scale. *Acta Psychiatrica Scandinavica* 1983; 67: 361–70.
5. Gilbody SM, House AO, Sheldon TA. Routinely administered questionnaires for depression and anxiety: systematic review. *BMJ* 2001; 322: 406–409.
6. Beck AT, Ward CH, Mendelson M, Mock J, Erbaugh J. An inventory for measuring depression. *Archives of General Psychiatry* 1961; 4: 561–71.
7. Lowe B, Unutzer J, Callahan CM, Perkins AJ, Kroenke K. Monitoring depression treatment outcomes with the patient health questionnaire-9. *Medical Care* 2004; 42: 1194–201.
8. Endicott J. Measurement of depression in patients with cancer. *Cancer* 1984; 53: 2243–9.
9. Burvill PW, Johnson GA, Jamrozik KD, Anderson CS, Stewart-Wynne EG, Chakera TM. Prevalence of depression after stroke: the Perth Community Stroke Study. *British Journal of Psychiatry* 1995; 166: 320–7.
10. Robinson RG. Poststroke depression: prevalence, diagnosis, treatment and disease progression. *Biological Psychiatry* 2003; 54: 376–87.

11. House A, Knapp P, Bamford J, Vail A. Mortality at 12 and 24 months after stroke may be associated with depressive symptoms at 1 month. *Stroke* 2001; 32: 696–701.

12. Carson AJ, MacHale S, Allen K et al. Depression after stroke and lesion location: a systematic review. *Lancet* 2000; 356: 122–6.

13. Narushima K, Paradiso S, Moser DJ, Jorge R, Robinson R. Effect of antidepressant therapy on executive function after stroke. *British Journal of Psychiatry* 2007; 190: 260–5.

14. Frasure-Smith N, Lespérance F, Talajic M. Depression following myocardial infarction: impact on 6-month survival. *Journal of the American Medical Association* 1993; 270: 1819–25.

15. Glassman AH, O'Connor CM, Califf RM et al., for the Sertraline Antidepressant Heart Attack Randomized Trial (SADHART) Group. Sertraline treatment of major depression in patients with acute MI or unstable angina. *Journal of the American Medical Association* 2002; 288: 701–709.

16. Carney RM, Blumenthal JA, Freedland KE et al.; ENRICHD Investigators. Depression and late mortality after myocardial infarction in the Enhancing Recovery in Coronary Heart Disease (ENRICHD) study. *Psychosomatic Medicine* 2004; 66: 466–74.

17. Lespérance F, Frasure-Smith N, Koszycki D et al., for the CREATE Investigators. Effects of citalopram and interpersonal psychotherapy on depression in patients with coronary artery disease. The Canadian Cardiac Randomized Evaluation of Antidepressant and Psychotherapy Efficacy (CREATE) Trial. *Journal of the American Medical Association* 2007; 297: 367–79.

18. Schrag A, Jahanshahi M, Quinn N. What contributes to the quality of life in patients with Parkinson's disease? *Journal of Neurology Neurosurgery and Psychiatry* 2000; 69: 308–12.

19. Sharpe M, Strong V, Allen K et al. Management of major depression in outpatients attending a cancer centre: a preliminary evaluation of a multicomponent cancer nurse-delivered intervention. *British Journal of Cancer* 2004; 90: 310–13.

20. Holland JC, Rowland J, Lebovits A Rusalem R. Reactions to cancer treatment: assessment of emotional response to adjunct radiotherapy. *Psychiatric Clinics of North America* 1979; 2: 347–58.

21. Moorey S, Greer S. *Cognitive Behaviour Therapy for People with Cancer.* Oxford: Oxford University Press; 2002.

22. Himelhoch S, Medoff DR. Efficacy of antidepressant medication among HIV-positive individuals with depression: a systematic review and meta-analysis. *AIDS Patient Care and STDs* 2005; 19: 813–22.

23. Markowitz JC, Kocsis JH, Fishman B et al. Treatment of depressive symptoms in human immunodeficiency virus-positive patients. *Archives of General Psychiatry* 1998; 55: 452–7.

24. Nixon S, O'Brien K, Glazier RH, Tynan AM. Aerobic exercise interventions for adults living with HIV/AIDS. *Cochrane Database of Systematic Reviews* 2002; (2): CD001796.

25. Gill D, Hatcher S. A systematic review of the treatment of depression with antidepressant drugs in patients who also have a physical illness. *Journal of Psychosomatic Research* 1999; 47: 131–43.

26. Sharpe L, Sensky T, Timberlake N, Ryan B, Brewin CR, Allard S. A blind, randomized, controlled trial of cognitive-behavioural intervention for patients with recent onset rheumatoid arthritis: preventing psychological and physical morbidity. *Pain* 2001; 89: 275–83.

27. de Mello FM, de Jesus Mari J, Bacaltchuk J, Verdeli H, Neugebauer R. A systematic review of research findings on the efficacy of interpersonal therapy for depressive disorders. *European Archives of Psychiatry and Clinical Neuroscience* 2005; 255: 75–82.

28. Antoni MH, Lehman JM, Kilbourn KM Boyers, A E; Culver, J L; Alferi, S M Yount, S E; McGregor, B A; Arena, P L; Harris, S D; Price, A; Carver, C S;. Cognitive-behavioral stress management intervention decreases the prevalence of depression and enhances benefit finding among women under treatment for early-stage breast cancer. *Health Psychology* 2001; 20: 20–32.

29. Sharpe L, Sensky T, Timberlake N, Ryan B, Brewin CR, Allard S. A blind, randomized, controlled trial of cognitive-behavioural intervention for patients with recent onset rheumatoid arthritis: preventing psychological and physical morbidity. *Pain* 2001; 89: 275–83.

10

Physical Consequences of Eating Disorders

Kate Webb, J. Hubert Lacey and John Morgan

The first important descriptions of anorexia nervosa came in the late 19th century by William Gull and Charles Lasegue, although case histories for people with probable anorexia nervosa had been reported long before. However, it was through authors such as Hilde Bruch, Arthur Crisp and Gerald Russell, that we have the modern concept of the disorder. The binge–purge subtype for anorexia nervosa was subsequently described and became a common presentation for the disorder. Bulimia nervosa was then described and named in 1979 by Gerald Russell and was incorporated into the ICD-10 *Classification of Mental and Behavioural Disorders* (ICD-10)[1] and the *Diagnostic and Statistical Manual of Mental Disorders*, third revised and fourth edition (DSM-III-R and IV). Multi-impulsive eating disorders and disorders classified under 'eating disorders not otherwise specified' (EDNOS) in DSM-IV, including disorders such as 'binge-eating disorder', 'purging disorder' and 'partial syndrome anorexia or bulimia nervosa' are being increasingly described.

Eating disorders are common and carry one of the highest standardised mortality rates of any psychiatric disorder and among the highest rates of disability. Physical complications are common in all eating disorders but anorexia nervosa carries the most serious physical risk. The management of patients with severe anorexia nervosa can raise significant anxieties for all involved in their care. Of particular concern are patients who are ambivalent or actively resistant to treatment, but who are deteriorating physically.

Initial physical examination and investigations

Many patients with an eating disorder will present to their general practitioner in the first instance and therefore initial diagnosis, and psychological and physical risk assessment, will be carried out in primary care, before referral on to general psychiatry or specialist eating disorders services. However, physical complications of eating disorders, particularly anorexia nervosa, affect every organ system in the body and patients may find themselves in other specialist clinics, such as cardiology, neurology, gastroenterology, endocrinology, gynaecology or dental surgeries, before an eating disorder is recognised. Although organic causes for unexplained weight loss should always be excluded and patients may have comorbid physical illness, either as a consequence of or unrelated to the eating disorder, compounding physical risk, it is clearly incumbent upon clinicians from all specialties to have an adequate knowledge of eating disorders, to recognise probable cases, and to refer to eating disorders services appropriately (Figure 10.1).

The decision to refer to general psychiatric services or specialist eating disorders services will depend on the availability of services and the local referral policies. The severity of the patients' physical status will usually determine the urgency of the referral and, occasionally, an emergency admission to a medical ward will be required at any stage of the referral, assessment and treatment process.

Initial physical assessment should include:

1. general medical, gynaecological and surgical history
2. general physical examination including cardiovascular, respiratory, abdominal, neurological, oral and dermatological examination
3. body mass index (BMI) = weight (kilograms)/height^2 (metres^2)
4. examination for proximal myopathy – e.g. sit-up or squat test
5. blood tests – full blood count (FBC); urea, creatinine, electrolytes including sodium, potassium, chloride, bicarbonate, phosphate and magnesium; liver function tests (LFTs) and glucose.
6. thyroid function tests (TFTs) and erythrocyte sedimentation rate (ESR) should be considered but are not a mandatory part of the initial risk assessment
7. core temperature
8. blood pressure (lying and standing) and pulse rate
9. electrocardiogram (ECG).

Investigations should be repeated regularly and when necessary and physical risk assessment should be seen as a longitudinal process.

The responsibility for physical monitoring until referral will usually lie with the general practitioner in primary care. Following referral and acceptance of the patient by a specialist eating disorders service, the

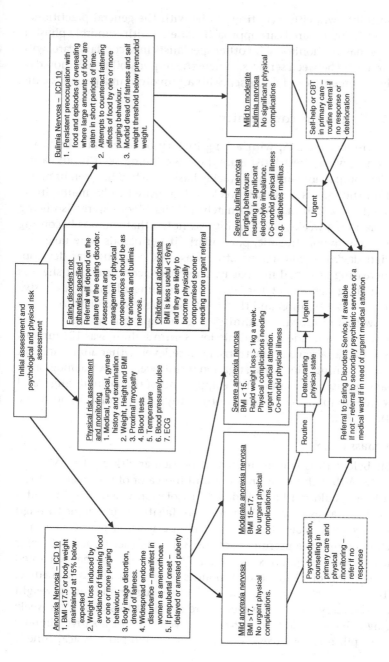

Figure 10.1 Algorithm for referral[2]

Note: BMI = body mass index; ECG = electrocardiogram; CBT = cognitive-behavioural therapy.

Anorexia Nervosa – ICD 10
1. BMI <17.5 or body weight maintained at 15% below expected
2. Weight loss induced by avoidance of fattening food or one or more purging behaviour.
3. Body image distortion, dread of fatness.
4. Widespread endocrine disturbance – manifest in women as amenorrhoea.
5. If prepubertal onset – delayed or arrested puberty

Bulimia Nervosa – ICD 10
1. Persistent preoccupation with food and episodes of overeating where large amounts of food are eaten in short periods of time.
2. Attempts to counteract fattening effects of food by one or more purging behaviour.
3. Morbid dread of fatness and self weight threshold below premorbid weight.

Initial assessment and psychological and physical risk assessment

Eating disorders not otherwise specified – Referral will depend on the nature of the eating disorder. Assessment and management of physical consequences should be as for anorexia and bulimia nervosa.

Physical risk assessment and monitoring
1. Medical, surgical, gynae history and examination.
2. Weight, Height and BMI
3. Proximal myopathy
4. Blood tests
5. Temperature
6. Blood pressure/pulse
7. ECG

Children and adolescents BMI is less useful <16yrs and they are likely to become physically compromised sooner needing more urgent referral

Mild to moderate bulimia nervosa No significant physical complications

Severe bulimia nervosa Purging behaviours resulting in significant electrolyte imbalance. Co-morbid physical illness e.g. diabetes melitus.

Self-help or CBT in primary care – routine referral if no response or deterioration

Urgent

Mild anorexia nervosa BMI >17. No urgent physical complications.

Moderate anorexia nervosa BMI 15–17. No urgent physical complications.

Severe anorexia nervosa BMI < 15. Rapid weight loss > 1kg a week. Physical complications needing urgent medical attention. Co-morbid physical illness

Psychoeducation, counselling in primary care and physical monitoring – refer if no response

Routine

Deteriorating physical state

Urgent

Referral to Eating Disorders Service, if available If not – referral to secondary psychiatric services or a medical ward if in need of urgent medical attention responsibility will either continue to lie with the general practitioner, or there may be a shared care approach. Patients with comorbid physical illnesses may be monitored by other specialists in secondary care, with regular liaison between services. Where the responsibility lies should be clearly documented and discussed with all involved in a patient's care.

Monitoring in the community

A 39-year-old female JS, with a long history of severe and enduring anorexia nervosa – restrictive subtype – was being seen in an eating disorders outpatient clinic on a weekly basis. She had her weight monitored on the same scales each week and appeared to be maintaining her weight at a BMI of approximately 14. Her bloods were also being monitored on a weekly basis and it was noted that she was becoming increasingly hyponatraemic, particularly if her bloods were taken on a 'weigh day'. Her core temperature was 35°C and she was developing increasing proximal myopathy. There were concerns that she was manipulating her weight through water loading (drinking excessive water prior to weighing) and that her true weight was likely to be 3–4 kg below that recorded. An admission to an inpatient eating disorders ward was recommended. On admission, serum sodium was 121 mmol/l and she had a raised alanine transaminase level. Other abnormal, but not as concerning, blood investigation results were a low haemoglobin, a mean corpuscular volume at the upper end of the normal range, and a low free thyroxine (T_4) with a normal thyroid-stimulating hormone (TSH).

Body mass index

A BMI below 15 is concerning, with particular risk as the BMI falls below 13. Although BMI is an important indicator of the level of physical risk, it should not be considered in isolation when carrying out a physical risk assessment.[3,4] Patients may falsify their weight through methods such as water loading or carrying weights in their clothes, which may limit the usefulness of the BMI. Another important factor is the rapidity of weight loss, for example, a patient who has remained stable at a BMI of 12 for several months or years, is at less immediate risk than a patient who is at a BMI of 14 through rapid recent weight loss. Particularly concerning factors are a weight loss of >1 kg a week; purging behaviours such as self-induced vomiting or laxative, diuretic and diet pill misuse; excessive exercise; or comorbid physical illness, such as insulin-dependent diabetes mellitus. BMI is also less useful in children and adolescents, in pregnancy, and in people with heights at the extremes of the normal range.

Proximal myopathy

Proximal myopathy occurs in patients with anorexia nervosa, due to starvation and the breakdown of muscle for energy. It can be assessed by asking the patient to lie on the floor or couch and attempting to sit up without using their hands for leverage or balance (sit-up test), or asking the patient to stand up from a squat position, again without using their hands for leverage or balance (squat test). With increasing emaciation, a patient will find these more of a struggle and this may be a better indicator of weight loss than BMI in a patient who manipulates their weight in some way.[3,4]

Blood tests

Full blood count

Mild anaemia is more common in patients with severe restrictive anorexia nervosa than in the general population. The prevalence has perhaps been underestimated due to haemoconcentration in a starved and dehydrated patient, meaning that anaemia may not become apparent until a patient starts refeeding. Anaemia is usually normocytic in these patients, but the mean corpuscular volume tends to be at the higher end of the normal range, and macrocytosis without anaemia is also common. Morphological changes to red cells in anorexia nervosa have been reported, particularly anthrocytosis, which has been attributed to lipoprotein changes and results in a low ESR. Patients with anorexia nervosa, especially as weight loss becomes more severe, often have a low white cell count, particularly neutropenia, which is perhaps the most concerning haematological abnormality in anorexia nervosa. There has been debate in the literature about the link between neutropenia and the occurrence of severe infection. It has also been suggested that infection in these patients is related not only to white cell changes, but also to other abnormalities in the immune system associated with starvation. Mild thrombocytopenia may occur in anorexia nervosa but consequent purpura is rare. Bone marrow changes would appear to have a pivotal role in haematological complications in patients with anorexia nervosa, due to fat cell depletion, which has a marked effect on haemopoiesis.[5]

Urea, creatinine and electrolytes

Eating disorders commonly cause problems with renal function, particularly related to dehydration due to reduced fluid intake or purging. Other conditions, such as rhabdomyolysis as a result of hypokalaemia, may cause acute and chronic renal failure.

Chronic and excessive vomiting usually causes a hypokalaemic, hypochloraemic metabolic alkalosis, with a normal, decreased or increased sodium. Laxative and diuretic misuse may also cause hypokalaemia with varying disturbances of pH, sodium and chloride. Hypokalaemia is a particularly concerning electrolyte disturbance and can result in cardiac arrhythmias, renal and gastrointestinal disturbances, muscle weakness, cramps, tetany and absent reflexes.[6] Oral supplements such as Sando-K® can be used, but if the serum potassium is <3 mmol/l, particularly if this is with associated ECG changes, a medical admission for rehydration and restoration of electrolytes may be necessary.

Hypophosphataemia, hypomagnesaemia and hypocalcaemia are associated with severe malnutrition, purging behaviours and alcohol misuse, and may also fall precipitously as a feature of refeeding syndrome (see below).

'Water loading' to manipulate weight can also cause hyponatraemia. In severe cases this can cause symptoms of 'water intoxication', including ataxia, confusion, seizures, coma and death, as a result of cerebral oedema and brainstem coning.[7]

Patients who purge are usually hypovolaemic, activating the angiotensin-renin-aldosterone system. If a patient suddenly stops purging, they may develop rebound oedema. This sometimes causes rapid weight gain, which will usually settle over a couple of weeks with conservative management including leg elevation. A potassium-sparing diuretic may very occasionally be used in the short term, if the oedema is persistent or particularly distressing for the patient.[8]

Glucose

Severe malnutrition can result in hypoglycaemia. This is often asymptomatic in patients with anorexia nervosa but may produce clinical symptoms and, in severe cases, hypoglycaemic coma and death. 'Dumping syndrome', where excessive insulin is produced in response to a meal, may occur during refeeding. Vomiting after bingeing in anorexia or bulimia nervosa can also cause hypoglycaemia and may perpetuate the binge–purge cycle, as bingeing will alleviate hypoglycaemia.[6]

Liver function tests

LFTs can become abnormal during starvation. This is thought to be related to fatty infiltration of the liver,[9] causing a mild hepatitic picture. Refeeding in patients with anorexia nervosa may also cause mild to moderate LFT abnormalities that should improve with further refeeding. Alcohol misuse in patients with eating disorders and abnormal LFTs should also be considered.

Albumin

A low serum albumin, indicative of severe and chronic starvation and/ or severe infection, is a strong predictor of death in anorexia nervosa, alongside severity of weight loss.[10,11]

Endocrine tests

Thyroid function tests are useful as part of an initial screen to rule out thyroid dysfunction as a comorbid illness, or to identify misuse of thyroxine. The thyroid axis is affected by eating disorders, particularly anorexia nervosa, but sometimes bulimia nervosa, and the usual pattern is a reduced tri-iodothyronine (T_3) and a normal TSH. T_4 may also be reduced in anorexia nervosa. Abnormalities directly related to the eating disorder should return to normal with weight gain and will not routinely need treatment. Other endocrine abnormalities that may occur are increased growth hormone and increased cortisol with normal or reduced adrenocorticotrophic hormone (ACTH). These do not need to be measured routinely unless there is concern about conditions such as Addison's disease as a differential for anorexia nervosa.[6] A reproductive hormonal profile may be necessary if a patient has not menstruated after a few months following weight restoration.

Core temperature

A low core temperature is common in anorexia nervosa, due to a poor autonomic response to temperature change. A temperature of <34.5°C is a concerning feature, indicative of serious physical risk.

RG, a 25-year-old woman, was admitted to an eating disorders ward with a diagnosis of anorexia nervosa, binge–purge subtype. Her main purging behaviour was vomiting. She had had a few admissions to a medical ward due to dehydration and electrolyte imbalance over the previous 6 months, and was not able to use outpatient care in an eating disorders service in a beneficial way. On admission, her BMI was 15 and had been falling for the previous 2 months. Her blood pressure was

90/65 mmHg lying and 70/50 mmHg standing. Her pulse was regular at 38 beats per minute and her ECG showed a prolonged QTc interval at 486 ms. Abnormal blood results revealed a low serum potassium, and a slightly raised urea. In this case, the postural drop and high urea suggested hypovolaemia, most likely as a result of vomiting, due to the specific electrolyte disturbances. Although a moderately raised urea and a postural drop in blood pressure would not cause immediate concern in themselves, rapid weight loss and the very low potassium resulting in a prolonged QTc and bradycardia, would need urgent attention due to the risk of fatal arrhythmias.

Blood pressure

Postural hypotension is common in patients with eating disorders, particularly those who are starved or hypovolaemic due to purging or fluid restriction, and blood pressure should be routinely monitored. Blood pressure <90/70 mmHg and a postural drop of >10 mmHg are concerning.[4]

ECG

Prolonged QTc interval

The QT interval represents ventricular depolarisation and repolarisation. QTc is the QT interval corrected for heart rate. Prolongation of the QTc interval and QT variability are two of the best predictors of potential life-threatening ventricular arrhythmias that can result in sudden cardiac death. The normal range is variable, but generally a QTc interval of >440 ms is thought of as abnormal. The QTc interval can be affected by many factors in a patient with an eating disorder, including starvation and low BMI, and purging behaviours and the resulting electrolyte abnormalities, particularly hypokalaemia and hypomagnesaemia. Prolonged starvation can cause atrophy and histological changes in cardiac muscle and collagen fibres. This and/or electrolyte imbalances may adversely affect cardiac electrophysiology, which can either be directly arrhythmiagenic or result in a prolonged QTc interval, predisposing the patient to potentially fatal ventricular arrhythmias.[12,13] A genetically prolonged QTc interval may compound the risk, as may some medications that can prolong the QTc interval, which should be used with care in patients with eating disorders.

Bradycardia

Bradycardia is common in patients with anorexia nervosa but concerning if <40 beats per minute, due to the risk of arrhythmias. A resting tachycardia is unusual in anorexia nervosa and should also be seen as a concerning feature, which may indicate severe infection or blood loss. It has been suggested that bradycardia in these patients may be due to an adaptive mechanism during starvation, to reduce cardiac effort caused by increased vagal tone. Thyroid dysfunction is also likely to be an adaptive mechanism to conserve energy and may be a contributory factor for bradycardia, as well as electrolyte disturbances, and atrophy and decreased glycogen content of cardiac tissue cells. Anorexia nervosa is associated with reduced variability of heart rate due to autonomic nervous system dysfunction. This is also thought to be a predictor of sudden death, particularly in patients with underlying cardiac disease.[12]

ST-segment and T-wave abnormalities

ST-segment and T-wave changes may suggest ischaemia and should be treated appropriately. These changes are usually related to starvation, hypothermia or electrolyte abnormalities and their effect on cardiac muscle.[3,13]

Echocardiography in patients with anorexia nervosa, will often show reduced left ventricular mass alongside reduced cardiac output. Other cardiac complications of eating disorders include mitral valve prolapse and pericardial effusion. Patients with bulimia nervosa who have ingested ipecacuanha as an emetic, are at high risk of developing toxic cardiomyopathy, which is potentially fatal.[12,13]

Most cardiac complications of eating disorders are reversible with weight gain, cessation of purging behaviours and restoration of electrolyte balance.

Admission

Most patients with eating disorders may be treated in an outpatient setting, either in primary care, secondary psychiatric services or tertiary specialist eating disorders services. Every patient should be monitored physically and risk assessment must be longitudinal. If there are particular concerns that monitoring cannot be managed on an outpatient basis, especially when there are significant electrolyte and cardiac disturbances, an admission to an eating disorders day hospital or inpatient ward should be considered. For patients at high immediate physical risk, many eating disorders units will be able to manage nasogastric tube feeding in patients who need urgent refeeding and are refusing an oral diet. Appropriate medical, dietetic and nursing support must be available and, if not, or if the medical complications are severe, an admission to a medical ward should be arranged. It is useful for eating disorders services to develop a good collaborative relationship with a consultant physician, who is prepared to manage patients with anorexia nervosa in emergency situations.

Refeeding and refeeding syndrome

NW, a 22-year-old Caucasian woman with a diagnosis of severe anorexia nervosa, binge–purge subtype, presented with rapid weight loss of 1–2 kg a week over 2 weeks. Her BMI has fallen to 11.5 and she was unable to stabilise her weight at home and therefore reluctantly agreed to a voluntary admission to a medical ward to start the refeeding process. Blood tests, including FBC, urea and electrolytes, LFTs, TFTs and glucose showed a low potassium, low chloride, raised bicarbonate and a slightly low free T_4. Her ECG showed a sinus bradycardia with a rate of 38 beats per minute and she had a low blood pressure of 85/60 mmHg, with a postural drop of 15 mmHg. A regime of bed rest and one-to-one nursing observations was instituted. An oral diet was initiated, under the guidance of the team dietician, to ensure a dietary regime that minimised the risk of severe refeeding syndrome. NW's serum phosphate levels decreased further after 2 days of refeeding, despite a low initial calorie input. Her cardiac state was monitored closely and she was given oral phosphate and potassium supplements, with daily blood monitoring, until her urea and electrolytes were stable and within the normal range.

Patients most at risk of refeeding syndrome are those with a BMI of <12, recent rapid weight loss of >1 kg a week, high alcohol intake, bingeing and purging behaviours, and comorbid physical illness.[10] Refeeding syndrome involves various electrolyte disturbances, the most important being hypophosphataemia. During starvation, endogenous stores are catabolised in order to provide energy, and insulin production is reduced, due to a lack of exogenous fuel intake. Intracellular electrolytes, in particular phosphate, are often depleted, even when serum levels are normal. On refeeding, particularly with a carbohydrate load, insulin production increases in response to the shift to exogenous carbohydrate metabolism. Insulin stimulates the uptake of electrolytes into cells, which may result in a precipitous drop in phosphate and other electrolytes. LFTs can also deteriorate on refeeding and should be monitored. Peripheral oedema may occur during refeeding and should be distinguished from cardiac failure. This may cause initial rapid weight gain but again usually settles with conservative management.

Blood tests should be monitored daily for at least the first 4 days of refeeding, and should continue if supplementation of electrolytes is needed, or until blood results are normal, when the frequency of blood tests can be reduced. Oral phosphate supplements can be used, or intravenous supplementation if the patient is on a medical ward and there is a severe drop in phosphate levels. Serum phosphate levels of <0.5 mmol/l can result in the clinical features of refeeding syndrome. These include rhabdomyolysis, acute haemolysis, respiratory failure, cardiac failure, hypotension, arrhythmias, seizures, coma and sudden death.[14] In order to minimise the risk or severity of refeeding syndrome, calorie intake in the first few days should be less than the patients' basal metabolic requirements and should be gradually built up. This will take careful supervision by a dietician, particularly for patients who are at high risk. Refeeding syndrome should not be forgotten for patients who are refeeding in an outpatient or day hospital setting, and there must be careful monitoring of diet and blood tests.

Compulsory refeeding

CH, a 22-year-old woman with a diagnosis of anorexia nervosa, was being treated as an outpatient by her local community mental health team. She continued to lose weight despite weekly input and physical monitoring by her general practitioner and persistently refused admission to a medical ward or a specialist eating disorders unit. Her team were divided about the use of mental health legislation, as some felt that to refeed against the will of the patient was a breach of human rights and that the patient had capacity to make a decision about her care. CH's weight fell to a BMI of 10.5 over a further 3 weeks and it was agreed that a Mental Health Act assessment should be arranged in the following few days. The patient was eventually detained on a medical ward, at a BMI of 9.8, but died of a myocardial infarction on the following day.

Compulsory treatment of patients with anorexia nervosa, involving compulsory refeeding, may be considered to be controversial but is not so in UK law. The Mental Health Act in England and Wales and associated case law, supported by coroners' statements, has clearly indicated the clinician's responsibility to ensure that the patient does not die. It is clearly preferable to develop and maintain a collaborative therapeutic alliance and for the patient to begin treatment through their own free will. However, there are times when a patient has become so seriously physically compromised, together with severe anorectic psychopathology, that they lack the capacity to make an informed decision in favour of life-saving treatment. Compulsory treatment may or may not temporarily upset the relationship between the clinician and patient but usually this can be rebuilt, perhaps with a stronger therapeutic relationship, in the knowledge that their illness has been taken seriously. The care plan can continue to be discussed and negotiated whilst the patient is detained under mental health legislation.

Use of the Mental Health Act should be considered proactively before it is too late to start the refeeding process and the patient is in life-threatening physical danger. Section 3 of the Mental Health Act 1983 (detention in hospital for up to 6 months for the treatment of a mental disorder) may be used in patients with anorexia nervosa for the purposes of refeeding, because the weight loss is a direct result of the core psychopathology that characterises the disorder.[15] Refeeding is life saving, and weight gain to a safer level may allow the patient to start working on psychological change, which will often not be possible during starvation due to cognitive deterioration. Children have fewer fat reserves than adults and will therefore usually reach a life-threatening physical state earlier, making intervention even more urgent.[10]

Refeeding under the Mental Health Act, against a patient's will, can be emotionally and physically arduous for nursing staff, and patients will require one-to-one nursing care. Control and restraint may be necessary and local or national guidelines for control and restraint of a severely agitated or violent patient should be adhered to, with appropriate and regular physical monitoring. Sedation, such as the use of lorazepam, may be necessary, taking body weight and cardiovascular and respiratory function into account when considering dosage. If there is concern about the physical safety of the patient, a medical admission should be considered, to start the refeeding process and to have access to more frequent physical monitoring and more accessible resuscitation facilities than might be available on an eating disorders ward in a mental health setting.

Other physical complications

Gynaecological problems

Anorexia nervosa and bulimia nervosa impinge on reproduction, both behaviourally and physiologically, with effects on menstruation, ovarian function, fertility, sexuality and pregnancy. Effects on fertility are some of the most important motivating factors for patients' recovery, as most changes are reversible upon recovery from an eating disorder.

Effects on menstruation include amenorrhoea, resulting from hypogonadotrophic hypogonadism in anorexia nervosa, and amenorrhoea or oligomenorrhoea, which occur in approximately half of patients with bulimia nervosa without loss of body mass. The ovaries of most patients with anorexia nervosa regress to a prepubertal state, hence the infertility in these patients, although this is usually reversed with weight restoration. Bulimia nervosa is associated with polycystic ovarian syndrome, although the causal relationship is unclear. This also leads to infertility and many patients with eating disorders may be found in infertility clinics.

Pregnancy is rare in anorexia nervosa and is associated with higher rates of spontaneous abortion, poor maternal weight gain and fetal growth retardation. Pregnancy in bulimia nervosa is not uncommon and is associated with being unplanned, either because of oligomenorrhoea and an assumption of infertility, or due to the association of bulimia nervosa and sexual impulsivity. Miscarriage, prematurity, hyperemesis gravidarum and fetal abnormalities are associated with bulimia nervosa. Eating-disordered symptoms may cease during pregnancy in patients with eating disorders, but many will relapse after childbirth.

Gynaecologists should be cautious in offering fertility treatments, such as artificial ovulation induction, to women with anorexia nervosa. Treatment for the eating disorder should be of primary importance. If pregnancy does occur in a patient with an eating disorder, particularly anorexia nervosa, careful monitoring of maternal nutrition and weight gain is important, as well as regular liaison between obstetric and eating disorders services.

Bone mineral density

Reduced bone mineral density is a significant complication of anorexia nervosa and is one of the few complications that is not completely reversible. Bone metabolism is a dynamic process where the actions of osteoblasts (cells that form bone) and osteoclasts (cells that resorb bone) work in conjunction with each other in a balanced way. Oestrogen normally inhibits specific cytokines that promote excessive bone resorption. Therefore, in patients with anorexia nervosa who are amenorrhoeic, excessive bone resorption, as well as a reduction of bone formation, contribute to the development of osteopenia or osteoporosis. Anorexia nervosa usually has an age of onset during teenage years, which is a peak time for bone mineral to be laid down. If this process is interrupted, the risk of reduced bone mineral density will be greater. There are other factors that are thought to be involved in the aetiology of osteoporosis or osteopenia in anorexia nervosa, as affected individuals tend to have lower bone densities than people of normal body weight who are amenorrhoeic for other reasons. These factors include a decreased level of insulin growth factor that normally stimulates bone formation, increased cortisol levels and other nutritional deficiencies.

Dual energy x-ray absorptiometry (DEXA) is usually used to measure bone density and has a relatively low radiation risk at approximately 10% of the radiation of a chest x-ray. Other than weight restoration, the evidence base for the management of osteoporosis in anorexia nervosa is poor and there are varying opinions about when DEXA scanning may be helpful during the course of the illness.

It would seem sensible to do a DEXA scan in all patients who have been amenorrhoeic for a year or more due to weight loss, as most loss of bone mineral density will occur after this time. Early scanning may be motivational in some patients, in terms of recovery. It may also be helpful for patients to know their bone density so that they can make informed decisions about lifestyle with knowledge of their fracture risk. Monitoring bone density through DEXA scanning every 2 years during recovery has been recommended, as significant changes to bone density are likely to take this length of time.

Weight restoration is the most important way of preventing deterioration and partly restoring bone mineral density. Exercise, particularly weight-bearing exercise, is known to improve bone density in a normal-weight individual, but strenuous exercise can also be detrimental to bone health in an emaciated patient, due to the increased fracture risk, the potential for increased weight loss, and continued loss of the menstrual cycle.

Bisphosphonates have a very poor evidence base for the treatment of anorexia-nervosa-related, premenopausal osteoporosis and should not be used in young women due to the potential side effects. They have adverse effects on the lining of the oesophagus and stomach and have also been shown to be teratogenic in animal studies, and remain bound to bone for several years. Hormone replacement therapy, the oral contraceptive pill (OCP) and calcium and vitamin D supplements are sometimes used routinely in patients with anorexia-nervosa-related osteoporosis but the evidence base for these treatments is poor. The withdrawal bleed that occurs with the use of the OCP may give the patient a spurious sense of health, which may be damaging in terms of motivation for recovery. Hormone replacement in children should be avoided due to the risk of premature closure of the epiphyses, causing stunted growth.[10,16]

Dermatological manifestations

Dermatological signs may suggest a diagnosis of an eating disorder. In anorexia nervosa, lanugo hair (hypertrichosis lanuginose) is very common and may be related to changes in thyroid function. It is manifest as soft 'downy' hair on the lower back, abdomen and forearms.[17] Russell's sign is common in patients with an eating disorder who self-induce vomiting by inserting their fingers into their throat to induce the gag reflex. This sign is due to the incisors causing abrasions and callouses on the dorsum of the hand. It often occurs near to the beginning of the illness, as patients who have induced vomiting for many years may be able to vomit without inducing the gag reflex. Other dermatological signs of eating disorders include carotenoderma, an orange tone to the skin caused by eating too many vegetables rich in carotene, and dryness of the skin, particularly in anorexia nervosa and probably due to a reduction in the activity of sebaceous glands, thyroid function disturbances and nutritional deficiencies. Acne may occur in anorexia nervosa, particularly during weight gain, and in bulimia nervosa associated with polycystic ovarian syndrome. Other dermatological problems that can occur include skin changes due to peripheral oedema during starvation or refeeding; changes to hair and nail structure, causing weakness and alopecia; acrocyanosis; and dermatitis. Patients who also self-harm may present with cigarette burns, scars from cutting, dermatitis from compulsive washing or picking of the skin and trichotillomania. Misuse of substances or purgative drugs may cause cutaneous drug reactions.[18]

Oral manifestations

Oral health can be significantly compromised in patients with eating disorders and may be most noticeable in patients who vomit. Enamel erosion is perhaps the most common oral manifestation. In patients who vomit, erosion will usually have a distinctive pattern on the lingual surface of the upper anterior teeth. Erosion is generally thought to take about 2 years to become clinically noticeable, although other factors such as the acidity of the patients' diet or differences in salivary pH or flow (reduced by some psychotropic medications), may alter the rate and patterns of erosion in patients with eating disorders, with or without vomiting. The research looking at dental caries in eating disorders is inconclusive, although it has been suggested that patients who vomit have a lower incidence of dental caries due to a lower pH environment in the mouth and better oral hygiene. When assessing dental caries in all patients with eating disorders, problems such as diet, vomiting and factors affecting salivary pH and flow, must be taken into account. Bone mineral density loss in patients with anorexia nervosa can worsen periodontal disease, as it means that a bacterial infection destroying alveolar bone will progress at a higher rate. Eating disorders can also cause problems with gingival and oral mucosal tissues through lack of oral hygiene, nutritional deficiencies, oral candidiasis and trauma from self-induced vomiting. Non-inflammatory hypertrophy of the salivary glands, particularly the parotids, can be found in patients who vomit. Self-induced vomiting also disturbs the gag reflex and abnormal swallow patterns have been shown in these patients.[19]

Any clinician assessing a patient with a probable eating disorder should ensure that they are aware of the oral health risks, particularly in patients who vomit. The aim of treatment should be to reduce eating disorder symptomatology, but simple advice concerning oral health can be given. This should include using a non-acid mouth wash or water to rinse after vomiting instead of brushing teeth immediately; limiting acidic foods and fluids; use of fluoride toothpastes; and regular dental appointments.[10]

Gastroenterological complications

Gastroenterological complaints are common in patients with all eating disorders, particularly those who binge and purge with self-induced vomiting or laxative misuse. In patients with anorexia nervosa, delayed gastric emptying may cause postprandial bloating, reflux symptoms and early satiety. Antiemetic medication, such as metoclopramide, speeds gastric emptying and may improve symptoms. Constipation is also a significant feature, often related to poor food intake and prolonged colonic transit. Constipation and delayed gastric emptying improve on resumption of a normal diet. Refeeding can, rarely, cause serious gastrointestinal complications such as acute gastric dilatation, rupture of the stomach and acute pancreatitis.[20] Hypokalaemia can also cause paralytic ileus or constipation.[6]

Self-induced vomiting can lead to oesophageal problems such as Mallory–Weiss tears, oesophagitis, hiatus hernias and reflux disease. Gastric dilatation and rupture due to bingeing, and oesophageal rupture due to vomiting, are rarer complications.[8] Haematemesis can be non-concerning or a medical emergency, depending on the cause, so must always be taken seriously. Patients with eating disorders are more prone to functional gastrointestinal disorders,[20] such as irritable bowel syndrome, and chronic laxative misuse may also resemble these disorders.[8]

Many patients misuse stimulant laxatives, and over time these can cause a breakdown of the colonic nerve supply and an atonic colon. Laxatives do not significantly reduce calorie absorption, which is counter to the common myth held by patients with eating disorders. However, they may cause dangerous abnormalities in electrolyte and fluid balance. In treatment, patients should be advised to wean off laxatives gradually to prevent rebound oedema. Regular food and fluid intake, and appropriate exercise, will also be helpful, although bulk laxatives may be required initially.[10] Investigation and treatment of gastrointestinal complications due to vomiting may be required.

Neurological complications

Proximal myopathy is probably the most common neurological complication of anorexia nervosa. Structural abnormalities of the brain, particularly widening of the sulci and ventricular enlargement, have been a consistent finding on neuroimaging in patients with anorexia nervosa. Most structural abnormalities appear to be reversible with weight gain, but some functional abnormalities remain, perhaps reflecting primary deficits. Electrolyte disturbances can result in various peripheral and central neurological complications. Vitamin deficiencies such as thiamine deficiency from malnutrition or alcohol misuse, may more rarely result in Wernicke's encephalopathy, and vitamin B_{12} and folic acid deficiency can potentially cause subacute combined degeneration of the spinal cord.[21]

Electrolytes should always be monitored and supplemented as necessary. It is usually only necessary to use a general multivitamin supplement during initial refeeding in patients with eating disorder.[10] More specific vitamin supplementation, such as with thiamine and vitamin B compound, may be required if there are clinical signs of Wernicke's encephalopathy, or evidence of comorbid alcohol misuse or severe and chronic malnutrition.

Other physical consequences

Other conditions such as diffuse soft tissue emphysema, superior mesenteric artery syndrome with associated acute gastric dilatation, kidney stones, chronic renal failure, rectal prolapse, severe tonsil hyperplasia related to vomiting, and central pontine myelinolysis associated with hypokalaemia, have been described in the literature as complications of eating disorders. These clearly reflect the diverse and serious nature of the physical consequences of eating disorders, which can affect all organ systems in the body.

Comorbid physical illness affecting physical risk in patients with eating disorders

Comorbid physical conditions, not directly a consequence of the eating disorder, are often associated with the development and maintenance of eating disorders and may compound the physical risk. Omission of insulin to effect weight loss in patients with diabetes mellitus may indicate an eating disorder and, in severe cases, will result in diabetic ketoacidosis, which is fatal without urgent medical treatment.[22] It has also been hypothesised that eating disorders may be a psychobiological defence against conditions such as cystic fibrosis, hypertrophic cardiomyopathy, Huntington's chorea and ulcerative colitis, which may worsen during adolescence, or for which pregnancy might be dangerous.[23]

Clearly, patients with comorbid physical illness should be followed up with the appropriate specialist team, in close liaison with the team treating the eating disorder.

Conclusions

Starvation, binge eating and purging affect all organ systems. The variables and manifestations are protean. Assessments must be repeated frequently. The physical management must be closely allied with motivational and supportive therapies. Great care should be exercised in the initial phases of refeeding. Active treatment should not be delayed, and if necessary should be provided under mental health legislation. Although many treatments can alleviate physiological distress, nothing is as effective as returning to a normal weight.

Key learning points

- Eating disorders, particularly anorexia nervosa, have a high morbidity and one of the highest standardised mortality rates of any psychiatric disorder.
- Longitudinal physical risk assessment is essential for all patients with eating disorders.
- Compulsory refeeding is a last resort but should be considered proactively as a life-saving measure.
- The dangers of refeeding syndrome are often not appreciated by doctors.
- Weight restoration is the primary treatment for physical consequences of eating disorders.

Key references

- Birmingham CL, Beumont P. *Medical Management of Eating Disorders – a practical handbook for healthcare professionals.* Cambridge: Cambridge University Press; 2004.
- National Institute for Health and Clinical Excellence. *Eating Disorders, Core Interventions in the Treatment and Management Of Anorexia Nervosa, Bulimia Nervosa and Other Related Eating Disorders.* Clinical guideline CG9. London: National Institute for Health and Clinical Excellence; 2004.
- Robinson PH. *Community Treatment of Eating Disorders.* Chichester: John Wiley and Sons Ltd; 2006.
- Treasure J. *A Guide to the Medical Risk Assessment for Eating Disorders.* London: Kings College London, University of London; 2004.

References

1. World Health Organization. *The ICD-10 Classification of Mental and Behavioural Disorders – clinical description and diagnostic guidelines.* Geneva: World Health Organization; 1992.
2. Royal College of Psychiatrists. *Primary Care Protocols for Common Mental Illnesses. Protocol III: Eating disorder (18+) – identification and referral.* http://www.rcpsych.ac.uk/pdf/pcProtocol.pdf (accessed 30 March 2011).
3. Robinson PH. *Community Treatment of Eating Disorders.* Chichester: John Wiley and Sons Ltd; 2006.
4. Treasure J. *A Guide to the Medical Risk Assessment for Eating Disorders.* London: Kings College London, University of London; 2004.
5. Lambert M, Boland B. Haematological complications. *European Eating Disorders Review* 2000; 8: 158–61.
6. Connan F, Lightman S, Treasure J. Biochemical and endocrine complications. *European Eating Disorders Review* 2000; 8: 144–57.
7. Rome ES, Ammerman S. Medical complications of eating disorders: an update. *Journal of Adolescent Health* 2003; 33(6): 418–26.
8. Lasater LM, Mehler PS. Medical complications of bulimia nervosa. *Eating Behaviors* 2001; 2(3): 279–92.
9. Winston AP, Gowers S, Jackson AA et al. *Guidelines for the Nutritional Management of Anorexia Nervosa.* Council report. London: Royal College of Psychiatrists; 2005.
10. National Institute for Health and Clinical Excellence. *Eating Disorders, Core Interventions in the Treatment and Management Of Anorexia Nervosa, Bulimia Nervosa and Other Related Eating Disorders.* Clinical guideline CG9. London: National Institute for Health and Clinical Excellence; 2004.
11. Herzog W, Deter HC, Fiehn W, Petzold E. Medical findings and predictors of long term physical outcome in anorexia nervosa: a prospective, 12-year follow-up study. *Psychological Medicine* 1997; 27: 269–79.
12. Casiero D, Frishman W. Cardiovascular complications of eating disorders. *Cardiology in Review* 2006; 14(5): 227–31.
13. McCallum K, Bermudez O, Ohlemeyer C, Tyson E, Portilla M, Ferdman B. How should the clinician evaluate and manage the cardiovascular complications of anorexia nervosa? *Eating Disorders* 2006; 14(1): 73–80.

14. Hearing SD. Refeeding syndrome. *BMJ* 2004; 328: 908–909.
15. Mental Health Act Commission Guidance Note, Guidance on the Treatment of Anorexia Nervosa under the Mental Health Act 1983. London: Care Quality Commission.
16. Mehler PS. Osteoporosis in anorexia nervosa: prevention and treatment. *International Journal of Eating Disorders* 2003; 33(2): 113–26.
17. Mitchell JE, Crow S. Medical complications of anorexia nervosa and bulimia nervosa. *Current Opinion in Psychiatry* 2006; 19(4): 438–43.
18. Strumia R. Bulimia and anorexia nervosa: cutaneous manifestations. *Journal of Cosmetic Dermatology* 2002; 1 (1): 30–4.
19. Frydrych AM, Davies GR, McDermott BM. Eating disorders and oral health: a review of the literature. *Australian Dental Journal* 2005; 50(1): 6–15.
20. Chial HJ, McAlpine DE, Camilleri M. Anorexia nervosa: manifestations and management for the gastroenterologist. *American Journal of Gastroenterology* 2002; 97(2): 255–69.
21. Chowdhury U, Lask B. Neurological correlates of eating disorders. *European Eating Disorders Review* 2000; 8: 126–33.
22. Crow SJ, Keel PK, Kendall D. Eating disorders and insulin dependent diabetes mellitus. *Psychosomatics* 1998; 39: 233–43.
23. Crisp, A. (2006), Death, survival and recovery in anorexia nervosa: a thirty five year study. *European Eating Disorders Review*, 14: 168–175.

Part III
Therapeutic Challenges

11

Neuroleptic-Induced Movement Disorders: Past and Present

Marie-Hélène Marion

In 1957, Delay and colleagues reported movement disorders in patients receiving chlorpromazine,[1] one year after treating the first patients, and recognised the similarity of these abnormal movements with those described in post-encephalitic parkinsonism (akathisia, orobuccolingual movements, tremor, oculogyric crisis and trismus). Since then, neuroleptics (NLs) have been widely used as there was no other alternative in the treatment of schizophrenia, and the extrapyramidal symptoms (EPS) became part of the unfortunate but unavoidable side effects.[2] Thirty years later, 'atypical neuroleptics' have decreased the frequency of these EPS, but they are still puzzling neurologists and psychiatrists as their physiopathology remains poorly understood and their treatment still far from efficient.

In this chapter we will review the clinical features of these EPS (Boxes 11.1 and 11.2), following a classification based on the chronology of their onset: acute dystonic reaction and acute akathisia, parkinsonism after chronic treatment, tardive dyskinesia (TD) and tardive dystonia persisting after discontinuation of the drug. Neuroleptic malignant syndrome is a rare and potentially fatal condition that can occur very early in the course of NL treatment, and will not be detailed in this chapter. Then we will consider what we have learnt since atypical NLs have been widely used, in terms of epidemiology and physiopathology, and discuss the therapeutic strategies, in particular the place of clozapine and of pallidal deep brain stimulation (DBS).

Clinical features

The diagnosis of EPS[3] can be easy if the patient reports a history of NL treatment or is referred from a psychiatrist, but can be more difficult if

---

Box 11.1   Neuroleptic-induced movement disorders that disappear after stopping the neuroleptic

Acute dystonic reaction: acute spasm of the jaw, tongue, larynx, pharynx or neck muscles with oculogyric crisis
Acute akathisia: distressing inner sense of restlessness, with inability to remain still and the urge to move
Parkinsonism: akineto-rigid or akineto-tremulous syndrome
Rabbit syndrome: fine, rapid rhythmic movement of the lips and jaw, but no tongue movement

---

Box 11.2   Neuroleptic-induced movement disorders that can persist after stopping the neuroleptic (tardive persistent movement disorders)

Tardive dyskinesia: orobuccolingual, truncal or distal limbs – rapid choreiform movements
Tardive dystonia: sustained dystonic spasms of the jaw, tongue, neck and paraspinal muscles associated with functional disability
Tardive tremor: 3 to 5 Hz, coarse and disabling tremor, predominantly postural, but can occur at rest
Tardive myoclonus
● *Tardive tics*

---

the patient is not aware of taking dopaminergic blockers (e.g. antiemetics, antidizziness medication, sleeping tablets and antimigraine tablets).

Acute dystonic reaction

Acute dystonic reaction (ADR) occurs in the first 5 days of starting a NL and usually has a fluctuating course. ADRs can be variable, depending on its severity, from a mild form with the feeling of a thick tongue, to a moderate form with transient trismus and torticollis, to a severe form with laryngo-pharyngospasm (the first episode of their sudden and brief occurrence is usually quite frightening for the patient). Commonly they present with jaw spasms, tongue protrusion, difficulty swallowing and tightness of the throat, abnormal head posture (torticollis or retrocollis) and rolling the eyes upward with deviation to the side (oculogyric crisis). There may be associated dystonic spasms of the arms, legs or trunk. They disappear following discontinuation of the dopaminergic blockers.

ADR should be considered in children or young adults who have been taking NLs or antiemetic drugs, such as prochlorperazine or metoclopramide, in the last few days. ADR is often misdiagnosed as malingering, hysteria or seizures. Young age (children and young adults) and gender (males are at two times higher risk than females) are the main risk factors for developing ADR. Dose of NL, particularly a very low or very high dose, is associated with less ADR than a moderate dose (about 400–1000 mg/day of haloperidol or its equivalent).

Acute akathisia

The term akathisia means the 'impossibility to remain seated'. It was first described in idiopathic and post-encephalitic parkinsonism. It is probably the commonest and most distressing movement disturbance associated with NLs,[4] and an important cause of poor drug compliance. Patients describe subjective experiences of inner tension, emotional unease, anxiety or, more specifically, the inability to remain still and the urge to move. The worst is standing still, for instance for queueing. Patients rock from foot to foot or tread on the spot; when sitting, they cross their legs repeatedly or swing their legs. In the more severe form, they are unable to maintain any position (tasikinesia). It occurs very quickly after starting or increasing the NL, it is dose dependent and improves with lowering the dose of NL. It occurs in approximately 20% of acute psychiatric admissions in patients receiving NL. Acute akathisia can progress to a chronic form and sometimes persist after discontinuation of neuroleptics (tardive akathisia).

Akathisia has some similarity with restless legs syndrome (RLS) but in RLS the urge to move occurs in the evening, is associated with marked dysesthesias and is relieved by walking. Psychotic patients often have difficulty communicating their feelings, and their descriptions can be misleading, resulting in a diagnosis of agitation or psychotic decompensation.

Parkinsonism

Neuroleptic-induced parkinsonism (NIP) was recognised quickly after the introduction of NLs and this was a major step in understanding the key role of the lack of dopamine in idiopathic Parkinson's disease (IPD). The prevalence estimates for NIP range from 5 to 50%,[5] and 90% of cases occur in the first 10 weeks of treatment. Most authors have found that advance age, pre-existing extrapyramidal signs or dementia,[5] and higher dosage of NL increased the risk of developing NIP, but a recent study has not found a relationship between NIP and duration of NL treatment or age of patient,[6] suggesting an individual predisposition to develop NIP.

All the cardinal features of IPD, rest tremor, akinesia, rigidity and loss of postural reflexes, can be present in NIP. A study comparing the clinical picture of NIP and IPD found symmetry of the signs in 61% of cases of NIP, a rest and action tremor in 44%, more pronounced parkinsonian signs in the upper limbs, mild gait disturbances and very rare freezing.[6] Although patients may develop incapacitating parkinsonism that can mimic catatonia, they are often unaware of the akinetic-rigid syndrome and are mainly aware of their tremor. IPD develops in up to 28% of elderly individuals with NIP,[5] reflecting an extra sensitivity of dopamine blockage in preclinical IPD.

The coexistence of NIP and TD[7] is about 17% and the presence of orobuccolingual dystonia in a patient with parkinsonism is the signature of a NL exposure. The bradykinesia should be distinguished from depression, psychological withdrawal or negative symptoms of schizophrenia. Hypokinetic features have also been described in catatonic schizophrenic patients, but they also present with particular awkward body positions that are maintained for a long period of time. In elderly patients it can be difficult to distinguish NIP from pre-existing IPD worsened by the NL and which will progress in the future. A history of slowness, walking difficulty or tremor prior to the treatment has to be searched for from the patient or his family. Dopamine transporter single proton emission computed tomography (DAT-SPECT) can be helpful to distinguish NIP from degenerative Parkinson's disease, as DAT-SPECT shows normal or increased DAT striatal activity in NIP.[8]

Rabbit syndrome is a fine, rapid, rhythmic lip and jaw movement, sparing the tongue, and which occurs during or after discontinuation of the NL treatment. It is a rare complication, which shares the physiopathology of parkinsonism and can be improved by anticholinergics.

Tardive dyskinesia

Spontaneous oral dyskinesias have been observed, particularly in elderly women, without any exposure to NL. Stereotypies (purposeless movements carried out in a repetitive way) and mannerisms (unusual ways of carrying out purposeful activities) can also occur spontaneously in schizophrenic patients and had been described well before the introduction of the NLs. Stereotypy and mannerism usually go together and result, for instance, in frowning eyes or blinking, lip smacking or grimacing, licking or protruding the tongue, head nodding, hand tapping or rubbing, rocking, hopping or skipping.

TDs are involuntary movements that occur following prolonged exposure to NL treatment (at least 3 months of NL drug treatment). TDs may occur during the NL treatment, at the time of the diminution of the NL dose, or at the discontinuation of the NL. TD may persist over

3 months after the discontinuation of the drugs (persisting TD). These tardive movement disorders are the most frequent drug-induced movement disorders referred to the neurologist and the most challenging in term of diagnosis and treatment.

The more frequent TDs are typically the bucco-linguo-masticatory dyskinesias, occurring in elderly women (Box 11.3) and are often ignored by the patient in the absence of functional difficulties (speaking and chewing are most often normal), but can be very difficult for the family to accept because of a grimacing appearance. Protruding, twisting, and curling tongue movements combined with lip and chewing jaw movements are characteristic. TD can also be more generalised in younger patients, with choreiform movement of the extremities (finger, foot, toes), abnormalities of gait and posture (rocking, swaying, lordosis, rotatory pelvic movement) and a grunting noise. They can be life threatening because of severe dysphagia or respiratory disturbances

Since the recognition of these TDs, many others have been described, such as tardive dystonia, tardive akathisia, tardive tremor, tardive tics and myoclonus.

Tardive dystonia

Tardive dystonia has been recognised more recently, and affects younger male patients (Box 11.4).[9] Although the majority have a focal craniocervical dystonia with blepharospasm, with or without oromandibular

---

Box 11.3 Risk factors associated with tardive dyskinesias

Older age
Female gender
Duration of exposure to neuroleptic
Duration of psychosis
Extrapyramidal signs
Family history of movement disorders
Cognitive deterioration
Anticholinergic preventive treatment
Use of typical NL

Box 11.4 Risk factors associated with acute and tardive dystonia

Younger age
Male gender
Family history of movement disorders
Use of typical neuroleptic

dystonia, retrocollis, antecollis or torticollis or axial dystonia, a less common initial presentation includes pharyngeal dystonia, tongue dystonia and laryngeal dystonia. Tardive dystonia tends to spread over the next 2 years to result in segmental or generalised dystonia. These dystonias are often very disabling (difficulty walking, chewing, speaking, swallowing or breathing) and sometimes painful for the patient.

Tardive dystonia of the jaw and tongue can be mistaken for TD, but the sustained jaw and tongue spasms, worse on action and responsible for difficulty speaking or eating, and the improvement with anticholinergic drugs are suggestive of dystonia.

Epidemiology of tardive dyskinesias

The risk of tardive dyskinesia

The risk of TD has clearly decreased since the 1990s, with the use of the second generation of NLs, also called atypical NLs.[2] The overall mean prevalence of TD among chronically treated patients with first-generation neuroleptic is 24%. Despite the remission of TD, chronic use of NLs appears to lead to a linear increase in the prevalence of TD (baseline 21%, after 5 years 38%, after 10 years 56%).[10] Randomised double blind comparison of the incidence of TD in patients with schizophrenia during long-term treatment with olanzapine versus haloperidol showed a decreased incidence with the atypical NL.[11] In the overall period, the 1-year risk of developing TD was 2.59% with olanzapine, compared to 8.02% with haloperidol, with a follow-up to 2.6 years. Interestingly in this large study, the patients who developed TD did not differ significantly from those who did not, with respect to baseline characteristics (sex, race, age, schizophrenia subtypes, duration of symptoms, positive or negative symptoms).

A recent systematic review of studies involving treatment with an atypical NL, lasting 1 year or more, gathering data on 2769 patients, has confirmed that atypical NLs have a reduced risk for TD, compared to typical NLs.[12] The weighed mean annual incidence of TD was 0.8% (range 0.0% to 1.5%) in the adults treated with an atypical NL compared to 5.4% (range 4.1% to 7.4%) in adults treated with haloperidol. In addition, a small study has looked at the incidence of TD in naïve drug patients with first-episode psychosis, receiving risperidone or haloperidol, and found 2 out of 229 patients on risperidone (0.87%) and 5 out of 215 patients on haloperidol (2.33%) developed TD, which was not statistically different, but it shows that TD can also occurs with an atypical NL.[13]

Also, since atypical NLs are more widely prescribed (Box 11.5),[14] particularly in vulnerable populations, such as children and the elderly with dementia, we need to be vigilant in the future about the incidence of side effects in these populations. As the prevention of TD is very important, factors such as a positive family history of movement disorders,[15] or the existence of extrapyramidal signs,[16] which may have a predictive value, also need to be taken in account before prescribing NLs.

The pharmacology of atypical neuroleptics

Blockage of the dopamine D_2 receptor with elevation of serum prolactin is the main action of the traditional antipsychotic drugs, and positron emission tomography (PET) studies in patients with schizophrenia showed that dopamine D_2 receptor binding is increased in long-term treatment with antipsychotics.[17]

Atypical NLs do not provoke catalepsy in animal models. One theory for their atypicality is blockage of the $5\text{-}HT_{2A}$ receptors at the same time as they block dopamine receptors (a serotonin–dopamine balance). A recent study in vitro and in vivo with PET scan suggests a 'fast-off-D_2' theory, with a transient occupation of the D_2 receptors and then a rapid dissociation to allow normal dopaminergic transmisssion.[18] For example, haloperidol remains constantly bound to D_2 receptors in humans undergoing two PET scans 24 hours apart, but the occupation of the D_2 receptors by clozapine or quetiapine has mostly disappeared after 24 hours.

Box 11.5   The most common conditions, other than schizophrenia, treated with atypical neuroleptics

● Psychosis associated with:
  – geriatric condition
  – dementia
  – Parkinson's disease
● Movement disorders
  – tardive dyskinesia
  – Tourette syndrome
  – Bipolar disorders
  – Obsessive-compulsive disorder
  – pervasive developmental disorders

Source: Adapted from Glick ID, Murray SR, Vasudevan P, Marder SR, Hu RJ. Treatment with atypical antipsychotics: new indications and new populations. *Journal of Psychiatric Research* 2001; 35(3): 187–91.[14]

Many pharmacogenetic studies[19] have also studied the association between polymorphism of cytochrome P450 (CYP) and TD.[19] Enzymes of the CYP family play a major role in the metabolism of NLs and therefore influence their efficacy and toxicity. In clinical practice, the identification of poor metabolisers by the knowledge of their CYP genotype could help with prescribing NLs outside toxic ranges.

Treatment

Treatment of EPS is difficult and the emphasis should be on prevention with careful prescription of NLs in high-risk patients and on early detection of the EPS.[20]

If a patient develops extrapyramidal side effects whilst taking an antipsychotic drug, ideal management is discontinuation or reduction of the antipsychotic drug, if this is psychiatrically feasible. Although parkinsonism and dyskinesia may disappear within several weeks, there is a potential to reoccur if the neuroleptic is reintroduced. If there is no other psychiatric alternative, and in particular in psychosis where the risk of relapse of the psychosis is high,[21] an atypical NL should be considered to treat the psychosis.

In addition, individual syndromes can benefit from symptomatic treatment as detailed next.

Acute dystonic reaction

ADR treatment is usually straightforward, with dramatic relief in about 15 minutes after parenteral administration of anticholinergics drugs. A second dose can be necessary in severe cases and oral anticholinergics should be continued for 48 hours in cases of early recurrence.

Acute akathisia

Anti-parkinsonian drugs such as anticholinergics and amantadine have been proposed but they are only partially effective. Benzodiazepines, in particular clonazepam (1 mg/day), have been studied in two randomised small clinical trials, with a reduction of the symptoms compared to placebo. The most promising treatment is with beta-blockers, with reduction of both the subjective and objective component of the acute akathisia in a double blind trial comparing propanolol (20–60 mg) to placebo.[22] Clonidine has also been studied, but the effect is limited by hypotension and sedation.

Parkinsonism

There are few controlled studies of the treatment of NIP with anti-parkinsonian drugs, and, in particular, the management is very difficult when NIP is associated with TDs, which are worsened with anti-parkinsonian drugs, particularly anticholinergics. Amantadine can have a transient benefit without increasing the TD. Levodopa is not the first-line treatment but can be proposed in young patients with parkinsonism. Electroconvulsive therapy (ECT) has also been reported to improve, transiently, both parkinsonism and TD.

Tardive dyskinesia and tardive dystonia

Treatment of TD is always difficult (Box 11.6). Although there are many published studies on the treatment of TD, relatively few treatments have proved to be consistently useful in practice.[20] There are no evidence-based data that show the efficacy of any drug in the treatment of TD. The emphasis should be on prevention and early detection of TD.

Review neuroleptic treatment

The therapeutic management is first to review the indications of the NL and try to stop it gradually if the patient is not schizophrenic. In the case of schizophrenia, a switch from a typical to an atypical NL should be discussed and if the patient is already on an atypical NL, a switch to clozapine should be proposed to the patient, with the implications of regular blood tests and the potential risk of agranulocytosis.

Box 11.6 Treatment of tardive dyskinesias

- Review the indications of the NL:
  - if not schizophrenia, try to stop the NL gradually
  - if schizophrenia, discuss atypical versus typical NL
- Confirm the nature of the movement disorder (dyskinetic versus dystonic):
  - in favour of a dyskinetic movement is presence of rapid movement of the tongue, no jaw spasm, no difficulty for speaking or chewing
- Stop anticholinergic drugs if present:
- After assessing disability, discuss with the patient:
  - trial of drugs (clonazepam, vitamin E, levetiracetam, cholinesterase inhibitors), which may help, but are not supported by evidence-based medicine data.
  - reintroduction of atypical NL, particularly clozapine
  - tetrabenazine
  - DBS surgery

Identify the movement disorder

Orobuccolingual dyskinesia should not be confused with jaw and tongue tardive dystonia, as the anticholinergic drugs may aggravate the dyskinesias (in contrast to tardive dystonia) and therefore should be stopped in the case of TDs.

In tardive dystonia, botulinum toxin is the most effective symptomatic treatment if the dystonia is focal.[23] Anticholinergic drugs and tetrabenazine[24] are the most useful drugs in the more generalised severe type and can be combined, but their efficacy is usually limited and the dystonia tends to persist (only 14% in the series reported by Kirikakis et al.[9] had a remission).

Mild tardive dyskinesia

In the case of mild TD, clonazepam, calcium channel blockers (diltiazem, nifedipine, nimodipine, verapamil), levetiracetam,[25] cholineresterase inhibitors and amantadine have been tried for treatment but there is no convincing double blind randomised study that shows the efficacy of these drugs.

Vitamin E, based on the rationale that TD may be due to free radicals, has been proposed, with mixed results.

Persistent and severe tardive dyskinesia

In some patients with persistent disabling dyskinesia, a NL can be reintroduced. All the atypical NLs have shown some efficacy in controlling TD, in particular the bucco-linguo-masticatory syndromes, in a range of doses lower than those likely to induce parkinsonian syndrome.

Tetrabenazine (50 to 200 mg) has a reserpine-like effect with a depletion of the presynaptic neurotransmitters.[24] It is used more by the neurologist than the psychiatrist, in severe TD and tardive dystonia. The main side effects, which are dose dependent, are hypotension, depression, akathisia and parkinsonism.

If the dyskinesias are very disabling, despite drug treatment, surgery has been proposed, in particular thalamotomy, pallidotomy and, more recently, bilateral pallidal DBS.[26] In a series of 10 patients with double blind evaluation, pallidal DBS was efficient in reducing the extrapyramidal score by a mean of 50%, without any psychiatric changes.

Conclusions

Thirty years after the description of NL-induced movement disorders, atypical neuroleptics, particularly clozapine, have been a major therapeutic advance for the prevention of these side effects. TDs have become rarer, but their physiopathology is still not fully elucidated and their treatment is still based on a strategy to alleviate the symptoms rather than on a cure.

Therefore we should be still vigilant; these movement disorders deserve all our attention and we hope that one day TD will become history.

Key learning points

- The incidence of tardive dyskinesias has decreased with the use of atypical NLs.
- Acute dystonic reaction can follow one dose of an antiemetic drug taken by a child or a young man and require parenteral anticholinergic treatment.
- DAT-SPECT is normal in the case of neuroleptic-induced parkinsonism.
- Involuntary oro-bucco-lingual movements in elderly people can be spontaneous, dyskinetic or dystonic in nature.
- Neuroleptic-induced movement disorders are psychologically, socially and functionally distressing and should be treated early and actively.

References

1. Delay J, Deniker P, Thuillier J. Similitude des accidents nerveux de la prochlorperazine avec certains troubles post-encephalitiques. *Annals of Medical Psychology* 1957; 1: 506–10.
2. Remington G. Tardive dyskinesia: eliminated, forgotten, or overshadowed? *Current Opinion in Psychiatry* 2007; 20: 131–7.
3. Casey DE. Neuroleptic-induced acute extrapyramidal syndromes and tardive dyskinesia. *Psychopharmacology*1993; 16: 589–611.
4. Adler LA, Angrist B, Reiter S, Rotrosen J. Neuroleptic -induced akathisia: a review. *Psychopharmacology* (Berlin)1989; 99(1): 134–5.
5. Caligiuri MP, Lacro JP, ParmD, Jeste DV. Incidence and predictors of drug-induced Parkinsonism in older psychiatric patients treated with very low doses of neuroleptics. *Journal of Clinical Psychopharmacology* 1999; 19: 322–8.
6. Hassin-Baer S, Sirota P, Korczyn Treves T A, Epstein B, Shabtai H, Martin T, Litvinjuk Y, Giladi N. Clinical characteristics of neuroleptic-induced parkinsonism. *Journal of Neural Transmission* 2001; 108: 1299–308.
7. Richardson MA, Craig TJ. The coexistence of parkinsonism-like symptoms and tardive dyskinesia. *American Journal of Psychiatry* 1982; 139: 341–3.
8. Scherfler C, Schwarz J, Antonini A et al. Role of DAT-SPECT in the diagnostic work up of Parkinsonism. *Movement Disorders* 2007; 22(9): 1229–38.
9. Kirikakis V, Bhatia KP, Quinn NP, Marsden CD. The natural history of tardive dystonia. A long term follow-up study of 107 cases. *Brain* 1998; 121: 2053–66.
10. Chouinard G, Annable L, Ross-Chouinard A. Fluphenazine enanthate and decanoate in the treatment of schizophrenic outpatients: extrapyramidal

symptoms and therapeutic effects. *American Journal of Psychiatry* 1982; 139: 312–18.

11. Tran PV, Dellva MA, Tollefson G Charles M Beasley, Jr., Janet H Potvin, and Gerilyn M Kiesler. Extrapyramidal symptoms and tolerability of Olanzapine versus Haloperidol in the acute treatment of schizophrenia. *Journal of Clinical Psychiatry* 1997; 58: 205–11.

12. Correll CU, Leucht S, Kane JM. Lower risk for tardive dyskinesia associated with second-generation antipsychotics: a systematic review of 1-year studies. *American Journal of Psychiatry* 2004; 161: 414–25.

13. Gharabawi GM, Bossie CA, Zhu Y. New-onset tardive dyskinesia in patients with first-episode psychosis receiving risperidone or haloperidol. *American Journal of Psychiatry* 2006; 163: 938–9.

14. Glick ID, Murray SR, Vasudevan P, Marder SR, Hu RJ. Treatment with atypical antipsychotics: new indications and new populations. *Journal of Psychiatric Research* 2001; 35(3): 187–91.

15. Lencer R, Eismann G, Kasten M et al. Family history of primary movement disorders as a predictor for neuroleptic-induced extrapyramidal symptoms. *British Journal of Psychiatry* 2004; 85: 465–71.

16. Tenback DE, van Harten PN, Slooff CJ, van Os J. Evidence that early extrapyramidal symptoms predict later tardive dyskinesia: a prospective analysis of 10,000 patients in the European Schizophrenia Outpatient Health Outcomes (SOHO) study. *American Journal of Psychiatry* 2006; 163: 1438–40.

17. Silvestri S, Seeman MV, Negrete JC, Houle S, Shammi C M, Remington G J, Kapur S, Zipursky R B, Wilson A A and Christensen B K, et al. Increased dopamine D2 receptor binding after long-term treatment with antipsychotics in humans: a clinical PET study. *Psychopharmacology* (Berlin) 2000; 152: 174–80.

18. Seeman P. Atypical antipsychotics: mechanism of action. *Canadian Journal of Psychiatry* 2002; 47: 27–38.

19. Bondy B, Spellmam I. Pharmacogenetics of antipsychotics: useful for the clinician? *Current Opinion in Psychiatry* 2007; 20: 126–30.

20. Tarsy D. Tardive dyskinesia. *Current Treatment Options in Neurology* 2000; 2: 205–14.

21. McGrath JJ, Soares KV. Neuroleptic reduction and/or cessation and neuroleptics as specific treatment of tardive dyskinesia. *Cochrane Database of Systematic Reviews* 2000; (2): CD000459.

22. Propranolol in the treatment of neuroleptic-induced akathisia (NIA) in schizophrenics: A double-blind, placebo-controlled study. Kramer, Mark S; Gorkin, Robert A; DiJohnson, Celeste; Sheves, Patricia *Biological Psychiatry*; Nov 1988; 24(7): 823–827.

23. Van Harten PN, Hovestadt A. Botulinum toxin as a treatment for tardive dyskinesia. *Movement Disorders* 2006; 21(8): 1276–7.

24. Jankovic J, Orman J. Tetrabenazine therapy of dystonia, chorea, tics and other dyskinesias. *Neurology* 1988; 38: 391–4.

25. Konitsiotis S, Pappa S, Mantas C, Mavreas V. Levetiracetam in tardive dyskinesia: an open label study. *Movement Disorders* 2006; 21(8): 1219–21.

26. Damier P, Thobois S, Witjas T et al.; French Stimulation for Tardive Dyskinesia (STARDYS) Study Group. Bilateral deep brain stimulation of the globus pallidus to treat tardive dyskinesia. *Archives of General Psychiatry* 2007; 64(2): 170–6.

12
The Clinician's Role in Helping Patients to Take Antidepressants as Prescribed

Alex J. Mitchell

Antidepressants are the most commonly prescribed medicine, accounting for over 100 million prescriptions per year in the United States of America (USA) alone, according to the Centers for Disease Control and Prevention. In accordance with national recommendations, they are often prescribed for periods of 6 or 12 months. Yet the advice given by prescribers, and the difficulties patients face taking medication for extended periods, have been poorly studied.[1-3] Most imagine it is relatively simple to follow a 5-day antibiotic course, but in reality only two-thirds manage to do so successfully.[4] Ask patients to follow a 7-day course, with antibiotics four times a day, and ideal concordance is achieved by only 39%.[5] As depression is increasingly thought of as a chronic illness, it is useful to compare medication habits with other long-term conditions.[6] Barber and colleagues (2004) found that only 16% of patients taking medication for stroke, coronary heart disease, asthma, diabetes and rheumatoid arthritis were adherent, problem free and in receipt of sufficient information when examined at 10 days.[7]

Should we expect our patients with mental health problems to be more or less able to adhere to our recommendations? Further, are we as clinicians prepared to change our (prescribing) behaviour in order to help patients with their (adherence) behaviour?

Nosology of difficulty taking prescribed medication

An understanding of why patients have difficulty taking medication as prescribed has advanced recently, with improved terminology for types of non-adherence (Figure 12.1). Whereas we previously talked

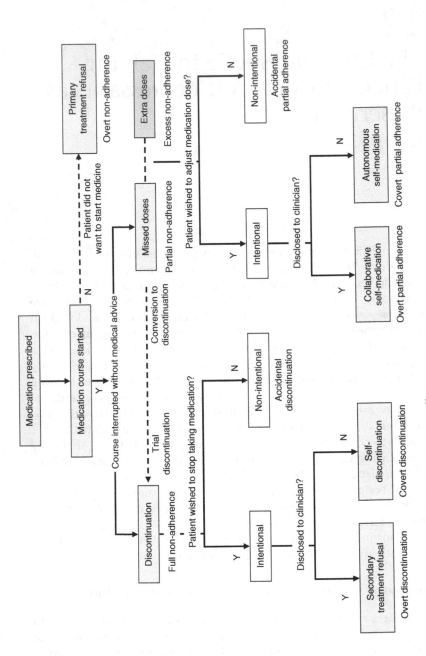

Figure 12.1 A new nosology of medication adherence

simplistically of compliant versus non-compliant, it is now recognised that there is a continuum of difficulty in relation to following medication advice. This continuum can be represented by the concepts of full and partial non-adherence as well as intentional and unintentional non-adherence.

A small proportion (10–20% in the case of antidepressants) of those prescribed a new drug will not collect the prescription and/or commence treatment. This is usually a reflection of an individual's uncertainty about the benefits versus hazards of that drug. Of those that do start, some take medication to excess, but, most commonly, occasional doses are omitted. This is called partial adherence and is extremely common, certainly more common that full discontinuation (see later). Not infrequently, patients miss doses intentionally due to inconvenience and also because of the belief that medication can be taken largely as required.

Doctors are not good at convincing patients to take medication for relapse prevention after the patient begins to feel better. For those taking medication long term, particularly those receiving little follow-up care, most will stop taking the medication themselves. They may or may not inform their doctor. Many will initially experiment with a period without medicine (trial discontinuation), after which they will either restart or decide to discontinue completely. Many of these decisions are entirely rational given the information available to the patient at that time. However, insight does play a role. Put another way, if someone does not perceive themselves as ill and is afraid of adverse effects, they are unlikely to put much effort into starting and continuing with a course of medication.

Epidemiology of antidepressant adherence

Several new studies suggest that adherence difficulties are common for patients who suffer from depression (see Box 12.1 for definitions). In the Medical Expenditure Panel Survey, Olfson and colleagues (2006) studied 829 people who had recently started antidepressant treatment for depression.[8] Forty-two% discontinued their antidepressants during the first 30 days and 72% had stopped within 90 days. Bambauer and colleagues (2006) documented partial non-adherence in 75% of depressed individuals, culminating in an average of 40% of days without dispensed antidepressants.[9]

In a prospective cohort study, Brook and colleagues in Amsterdam (2006) used 6-month follow-up data of 147 primary care patients who

---

Box 12.1   Types of poor medication adherence

Full discontinuation
Stopping a prescribed course of medication against medical advice (or in the absence of medical advice)

Partial non-adherence
Interrupting a prescribed course of medication against medical advice (or in the absence of medical advice)

Optimal adherence
Taking the prescribed medication, at the correct time and at the correct dose on a regular basis

---

were newly prescribed a non-tricyclic antidepressant.[10] Adherence behaviour was closely monitored using an electronic pill container, over a total equivalent of more than 20,000 days. The mean number of correct intakes was 74%, with 69% exhibiting adequate adherence (defined as taking more than 80% of medication doses). Remarkably, only 3% of the patients followed the medication regimen exactly as prescribed.

In a large national database study, Cantrell et al. (2006) conducted a retrospective study of patients recently prescribed selective serotonin reuptake inhibitor (SSRI) therapy for depression or anxiety.[11] On several measures of adherence, only 43% of patients were adherent to antidepressant therapy at 6 months. In a retrospective, observational study of 4312 depressed patients, Akincigil et al. (2007) measured treatment adherence using pharmacy refill records during the first 16 weeks (acute phase) of treatment and then up to 33 weeks (continuation phase).[12] Fifty-one% were adherent in the acute phase, and of those, only 42% remained adherent in the continuation phase. Low follow-up from a psychiatrist, younger age, comorbid alcohol or other substance abuse, comorbid cardiovascular/metabolic conditions, use of older-generation antidepressants, and residence in lower-income neighbourhoods were associated with lower acute-phase adherence.

Stein and colleagues (2007) examined antidepressant adherence in relation to anxiety disorders with or without depression.[13] In a sample of 13,085, 57% were non-adherent to antidepressant therapy at 6 months. Patients who received specialist mental health care were more likely to be adherent (48.5% versus 40.7%), as were those with dual diagnoses of anxiety and depression (46.8% versus anxiety alone – 40.2%).

These findings suggest that almost no one takes a long-term anti-depressant course exactly as directed, and premature discontinuation is the rule rather than the exception 6 months after starting a drug. This is line with previous studies. For example Tierney and colleagues found that of 240,604 patients who were given a new antidepressant prescription, 70% discontinued within 6 months.[14] In adherence data from over 740,000 newly initiated immediate-release SSRI patients, Eaddy and associates (2003) found that nearly 50% of patients failed to adhere to therapy for 60 days or more, and only 28% were compliant at 6 months.[15] These poor adherence figures represent real-world situations, as most have been collated from large healthcare databases. Further useful information comes from trial environments in which adherence is closely monitored and follow-up is extremely regular. Even here, discontinuation rates for those taking SSRIs are above 70%.[16]

Consequences of antidepressant non-adherence

There is considerable evidence that premature medication discontinuation can be costly.[17,18] Undisclosed (covert) non-adherence appears to be particularly hazardous, probably because alternatives are not explored. That said, in some cases non-adherence may be the sensible choice when current medication causes more harm than benefit. Thus, non-adherence may be costly, but this is not always the case. Unfortunately, there have been very few studies exploring the consequences of poor adherence to antidepressants or premature discontinuation of anti-depressants in clinical settings. Studies of relapse following planned discontinuation in trial environments illustrate high relapse rates but these may not be comparable to true patient-led discontinuation.

Recently Akerblad et al. (2007) studied the consequence of non-adherence in 835 patients followed for 2 years.[19] Response and remission rates were significantly higher in adherent compared to non-adherent patients. For example, 48.3% of adherent patients had a sustained response, compared with 25.4% of non-adherent patients. However, there was little difference in relapse rates, although the mean time from response to first sign of relapse was somewhat longer in the adherent patients (302 days versus 249 days).

Understanding discontinuation of antidepressants

What factors can explain these high rates of discontinuation and even higher rates of missed medication? Slowly, evidence is emerging that in the vast majority of cases, pre-existing treatment preferences, trust in medication/the prescriber, and treatment-emergent problems are more important than severity of depression or loss of insight (Box 12.2). In fact, most cases of discontinuation appear to be intentional and rational, given the information available to that individual. What does the research suggest about predictors of antidepressant non-adherence?

Confidence in antidepressant treatment

Sirey et al. (2001) found that perceptions of stigma about depression at the start of treatment predicted subsequent antidepressant adherence 3 months later.[20,21] Surveys in many countries consistently report that more than three-quarters of people believe that antidepressants are addictive, and most prefer psychological treatments or no treatment at all.[22–25] Col et al. found that 50% of depressed patients believed they did not need their antidepressants when they began to feel better, or that they could be taken 'as-required'.[26] Previous negative experiences of prescribed medication have a negative influence on current adherence behaviour.[27]

Box 12.2   Summary of predictors of missed antidepressant medication

External factors
- Lack of support
- Interruption of supply

Patient (intentional)
- Concerns about medication/stigma
- Concerns about cost
- Lack of efficacy

Patient (non-intentional)
- Cognitive impairment
- Complexity of regimen
- Distraction
- Loss of insight
- Misunderstanding instructions
- Previous negative experience

Healthcare professional-related factors
- Poor therapeutic alliance
- Poor empathy
- Little explanation about medication
- Inadequate follow-up
- Prescription of lengthy course

Indeed, Brook et al. (2006) found that attitude towards antidepressants was the most important predictor in determining reliable adherence behaviour.[10] Aikens and coworkers went further and modelled the risk attributable to concerns about medication.[28] Baseline scepticism about starting an antidepressant conferred a 62% increase in the risk of premature discontinuation over 9 months.

Effectiveness

In a large study of over 15,000 patients treated with fluoxetine in general practice, 33% stopped in the first 6 weeks; 64% stopped after feeling better, and 11% because of lack of response; 14% stopped because of tolerability issues.[29] Amongst 210 patients previously treated for depression who stopped medication, Ashton and coworkers (2005) found that the most common reason for discontinuation was lack of efficacy (reported by 44%).[30] However, many patients stop antidepressants intentionally, when they feel better. In fact, two studies found that one-third of patients stop by 3 months, citing feeling better as the reason, and 55% stop when feeling better by 6 months.[31,32] Thus, both successful and unsuccessful treatment often leads to patient-led discontinuation.

Adverse effects

Adverse events are an important but avoidable (or at least reversible) reason for discontinuing treatment and not wanting to restart. Ayalon et al. (2005) found that intentional non-adherence was associated with concerns about side effects of antidepressants as well as the associated stigma.[33] In a survey of 344 antidepressant users, the most common reason for less than perfect compliance was side effects.[30] The experience of one or more bothersome adverse effects means that an individual is three times more likely to stop medication.[34] Such complications include weight gain (31%), inability to have an erection (25%), difficulty reaching orgasm (24%) and fatigue (21%).[30]

Accidental omissions

If one examines missed doses rather than full discontinuation, then 'forgetting to take the tablet' is the most common explanation. This is encouraging as this allows scope for reminder systems (see later). In the large Alberta Mental Health Telephone Survey from Calgary, poor compliance was assessed in 5323 adults by the question 'When you take antidepressants, are there any days when you took less than you were supposed to'. Forty-two% of individuals missed medication and 64.9% reported that forgetfulness was the most common reason for missed medication.[35] Similarly, Ashton et al. found that difficulty remembering to take medication accounted for 43% of cases of poor compliance.[30] Forgetting to take all doses is related to regimen complexity, cognitive impairment, the duration of institutionalisation, and, ironically, the presence of depression.[36]

Choice of antidepressant

One obvious factor that deserves further comment is the effect of the specific antidepressant drug. Each pharmaceutical company claims superiority of tolerability but does this translate into differences in clinical practice? Surprisingly, robust differences in large-scale head-to-head studies are difficult to find. For example, work to date hints that discontinuation with tricyclics is only marginally worse than with newer antidepressants.[37-40] Similarly, differences between SSRIs, according to new data from 116,090 patients newly initiated on SSRI in the Integrated Healthcare Information Services (IHCIS) National Managed Care Database, are marginal.[41] Certainly, factors other than specific antidepressant choice seem to be the major determinants of partial non-adherence and premature discontinuation.

Measures to reduce antidepressant non-adherence

Collaborative care interventions

There are numerous potential ways of improving adherence behaviour, from simple to complex (Boxes 12.3 and 12.4).[42] Large-scale studies in medical settings suggest that dramatic effects on adherence behaviour are rare.[43] Mental healthcare studies have often examined a package of care, usually called 'collaborate care'. The collaboration is between mental health professionals and primary care practitioners. Key components may include patient education and support, monitoring of symptoms, psychological treatment options and help with treatment adherence. Several reviews of depression show benefits of collaborate care upon medication adherence, although individual differences between studies are large.[44,45] Collaborative care packages have demonstrated a benefit in 14 out of 28 studies that used adherence as an outcome (see Bower et al. for details).[46] However, disentangling each key component to discover which specific aspects help may be difficult or impossible. For this, other study designs are needed (see later).

Specific interventions

Only a few specific strategies have been rigorously tested in depression.[47-49] Vergouwen and colleagues (2003) reviewed six interventions conducted

Box 12.3   Basic strategies to enhance concordance

Basic communication/education

Establish a therapeutic relationship and trust
Establish patient concerns before prescribing
Take into account patient preferences for type of therapy
Explain the benefits and hazards of treatment options
Involve family members, if possible

Prescribing related

Simplify the timing, frequency, amount and dosage
Provide support, encouragement and follow-up
Consider blister/daily dosing pill boxes
Provide medication free or at reduced cost

Basic reminders

Send reminders via mail, email, or telephone
Increase home visits
Encourage family support

Evaluating adherence (basic)

Ask about problems with medication
Ask specifically about missed doses
Ask about thoughts of discontinuation

Box 12.4   Advanced strategies to improve concordance

Advanced reminders

Consider adherence aids, such as medication boxes and alarms

Evaluating adherence

Pill counting, measuring serum or urine drug levels
Electronic medication counting
Adherence questionnaires

Dispensing and drug administration

Consider a community health professional
Consider electronic dispensing aids

Psychological techniques

Compliance therapy
Insight therapy and cognitive-behavioural therapy (CBT)

Behavioural feedback

Reward high adherence with positive feedback

in mental health outpatients and 13 studies conducted in primary care.[50] Of those in psychiatric settings, five tested education as an adherence-enhancing intervention and three of these studies from Myers' group at the University of Keele could not demonstrate any appreciable effect.[51-53] However, Myers and Calvert[54] and Altamura and Mauri[55] both demonstrated significantly better adherence in patients who received verbal and/or written information about side effects of antidepressant medication. A recent review of simple strategies involving giving patients more information about their medication found 17 studies.[56] Generally, adherence was 11–30% higher in the intervention groups than in the control group. A combination of oral and written information seemed to have an added value, as compared to supplying exclusively oral or written information. However, no significant differences were seen for frequency of side effects, relapse or admission rates, symptoms and quality of life. Myers and Branthwaite (1992)[57] were the only group that tested the influence of the complexity of the frequency of dosing, as well as the effectiveness of allowing patients to choose their own dosage regimen. Adherence was significantly better in only those patients who were allowed to choose.

From the 13 primary care studies reviewed by Vergouwen and colleagues (2003),[50] three tested educational interventions but two involved a leaflet alone. None were successful at improving adherence.[58-60] Since early 2003, a further eight studies have been published (reviewed by Bower et al., 2006).[46] The largest was a randomised study involving 1031 depressed patients, which looked at an educational programme and therapeutic drug monitoring in those treated with sertraline for 24 weeks in primary care.[61] Here, Akerblad and colleagues (2003) found that neither of the interventions resulted in a significant increase in adherence rate. However, significantly more patients in the education group responded at week 24 compared to patients in the control group. In new study from Bambauer and colleagues in Boston, it was found that a simple intervention of faxed alerts regarding patient adherence was not successful in improving antidepressant adherence.[9]

The clinician's responsibility in promoting adherence

The finding that of all those who discontinue medication, 60% have not informed their doctor by 3 months, and one-quarter have not done so by 6 months,[31,32] should serve as a wake-up call to all prescribers about the importance of communication. All clinicians must maintain a high index of suspicion for possible treatment-emergent problems (adverse events and missed medication) but this should be communicated in a supportive rather than doubting manner. Simply discussing the *possibility* of an adverse event with the patient reduces the rate of unanticipated discontinuation by half. Similarly, the chance of discontinuation is about 60% lower in patients who are simply told to take medication for at least 6 months, compared with those who did not recall being given this information.[62]

Most patients with depression want to be involved in decision making.[63,64] Indeed, there is some evidence that adherence improves if more relevant information is given.[65] Yet analysis of doctor–patient discourses illustrates that clinicians ask approximately one in five patients how well their antidepressants are working, and only one in 10 patients if they are experiencing any side effects.[66] After analysing audio-recordings of interactions between 152 clinicians (internists and primary care) and patients, Young and coworkers (2006) discovered a mixed picture of communication.[67] Whereas drug purpose and side effects were usually mentioned, barriers to use and 'what to do if you missed a dose' were mentioned less than 2% of the time. Further, advice to continue to take the medicine even if feeling better, and advice to continue to take the medication until further review, were discussed on only 5.4% and 3.9% of the visits, respectively. Clinicians provided information about antidepressant treatment duration in 35% of interactions, which is interesting because Bull's group previously found that although 71% of clinicians claimed to specify treatment duration, 64% of patients recalled no such instructions.[34] This has led some to suggest it is practitioner behaviour that is the major remediable barrier to poor concordance.[68]

Brown and colleagues (2007) used the Patient Education Questionnaire[69] to measure clinician advice.[70] When measured by the percentage of prescribed doses taken, adherence was 82% at 1 month and 69% at 3 months. When measured by the percentage of days with correct intake and timing, adherence was only 55% at 1 month and 43% at 3 months. Several key messages about antidepressant medication differentiated adherent from non-adherent patients, including 'told what to do if there were questions', 'keep taking the medication even if feeling better', and 'told how long to expect to take medicine', 'advised of how long side effects will last', and 'given advice on managing minor side effects' (see Box 12.5). The odds of being adherent (measured by doses) more than tripled among those who said they were told 'how long to expect to take the medicine' and 'told what to do if there were questions', and the odds of being adherent (measured by days) doubled among patients who reported that they were 'told how long to expect

---

Box 12.5   Clinician advice when starting antidepressants

Do you have any concerns before starting antidepressants?
We only recommend medicine that we think will work
Start the antidepressant as soon as possible
Take the medication daily, even if you feel well
Expect the benefit to begin gradually, and not straight away
Mild side effects are common in the first week but usually wear off soon after this
Troublesome side effects are less common and can be helped
Please let us know if side effects develop
Most people take a first antidepressant course for 6 months
If this antidepressant does not work for you, we can try another
Please let us know how you are getting on in 2–4 weeks' time.

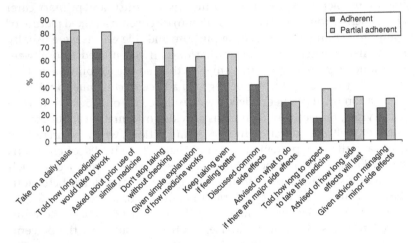

Figure 12.2   Frequency of clinician advice about starting antidepressants

Source: Adapted from Brown C, Battista DR, Sereika SM, Bruehlman RD, Dunbar-Jacob J, Thase ME. How can you improve antidepressant adherence? Talk to your patients about side effects and how long treatment will take. *Journal of Family Practice* 2007; 56(5): 356–63.[70]

to take the medicine' compared with those who said they had not been told.

Conclusions

Most, perhaps all, patients have difficulty taking medication for a long period of time. Depression management often necessitates taking antidepressants for 3, 6 or 12 months and occasionally, when the risks of relapse are very high, indefinitely. Viewed as part of the wide clinical process, difficulties with antidepressants include not only problems with efficacy and tolerability, but inadequate explanation upon starting the medicine and inadequate monitoring after starting. Recent evidence suggests that the majority of patients prescribed an antidepressant will experience some kind of problem that will lead to thoughts of discontinuation. Further, many miss doses due to simple lapses or inconvenience, and many will stop taking their medicine once they feel well. Although this may be associated with adverse outcomes in terms of relapse or readmission, missing doses and even stopping completely may be the most rational approach to health, given patients' understanding of their illness and the information available to them.[71,72]

Clinicians who are alert to these kinds of difficulties may prevent unmonitored discontinuation. Clinicians who are able to discuss the strengths and weaknesses of medicines and who appear to be open to feedback will foster greater trust and therapeutic alliance. At the same time, patients who have difficulty remembering to take their medication might be helped by simple reminder systems. Both partial non-adherence and discontinuation can be helped by enhanced collaborative care for depression.

Key learning points

Most people have difficulty taking medication exactly as prescribed for more than a week.

New antidepressants have significant adverse effects and are not always effective.

Antidepressants are only one possible therapeutic option for depressed patients.

Partial adherence is more common that full adherence.

Patients may stop or interrupt a medication course for rational reasons.

Clinicians should spend more time engaging patients in their depression care in a collaborative model.

Clinicians should discuss the advantages and disadvantages of all therapeutic options.

Patients may be helped to take medication more reliably using reminder systems.

Patient education and information promote adherence.

Collaborative depression care promotes adherence in primary care.

232   *Alex J. Mitchell*

References

1. Velligan DI, Weiden PJ. Interventions to improve adherence to antipsychotic medications. *Psychiatric Times* 2006; XXIII(9). http://www.psychiatrictimes.com/showArticle.jhtml?articleID=192202943
2. Mitchell AJ. High medication discontinuation rates in psychiatry: how often is it understandable? *Journal of Clinical Psychopharmacology* 2006; 26(2): 109–12.
3. Stein MB, Cantrell CR, Sokol MC, Eaddy MT, Shah MB. Antidepressant adherence and medical resource use among managed care patients with anxiety disorders. *Psychiatric Services* 2006; 57: 673–80.
4. Kardas P. Patient compliance with antibiotic treatment for respiratory tract infections. *Journal of Antimicrobial Chemotherapy* 2002; 49: 897–903.
5. Cheung R, Sullens CM, Seal D, Dickins J, Nicholson PW, Deshmukh AA, Denham MJ, Dobbs SM. The paradox of using a 7-day antibacterial course to treat urinary tract infections in the community. *British Journal of Clinical Pharmacology* 1988; 26: 391–8.
6. Andrews G. Should depression be managed as a chronic disease? *BMJ* 2001; 322: 419–21.
7. Barber N, Parsons J, Clifford S, Darracott R, Horne R. Patients' problems with new medication for chronic Patients' conditions. *Quality and Safety in Health Care* 2004; 13: 172–5.
8. Olfson M, Marcus SC, Tedeschi M, Wan GJ. Continuity of antidepressant treatment for adults with depression in the United States. *American Journal of Psychiatry* 2006; 163(1): 101–108.
9. Bambauer KZ, Adams AS, Zhang F, Minkoff N, Grande A, Weisblatt R, Soumerai SB, Ross-Degnan D. Physician alerts to increase antidepressant adherence – fax or fiction? *Archives of Internal Medicine* 2006; 166(5): 498–504.
10. Brook OH, van Hout HPJ, Stalman WAB, de Haan M. Nontricyclic antidepressants - Predictors of nonadherence. *Journal of Clinical Psychopharmacology* 2006; 26(6): 643–7.
11. Cantrell CR, Eaddy MT, Shah MB, Regan TS, Sokol MC. Methods for evaluating patient adherence to antidepressant therapy – a real-world comparison of adherence and economic outcomes. *Medical Care* 2006; 44(4): 300–303.
12. Akincigil A, Bowblis JR, Levin C, Walkup JT, Jan S, Crystal S. Adherence to antidepressant treatment among privately insured patients diagnosed with depression. *Medical Care* 2007; 45(4): 363–9.
13. Stein MB, Cantrell CR, Sokol MC, Eaddy MT, Shah MB. Antidepressant adherence and medical resource use among managed care patients with anxiety disorders. *Psychiatric Services* 2006; 57(5): 673–80.
14. Tierney R, Melfi CA, Signa W, Croghan TW. Antidepressant use and use patterns in naturalistic settings. *Drug Benefit Trends* 2000; 12(6): 7BH–12BH.
15. Eaddy M, Regan T. Real world 6-month immediate-release SSRIs non-adherence. *Program and Abstracts of the Disease Management Association of America 5th Annual Disease Management Leadership Forum*; 12–15 October 2003; Chicago, Illinois.
16. Mullins CD, Shaya FT, Meng FL, Wang JL, Harrison D. Persistence, switching, and discontinuation rates among patients receiving sertraline, paroxetine, and citalopram. *Pharmacotherapy* 2005; 25(5): 660–7.

17. Green JH. Frequent rehospitalization and noncompliance with treatment. *Hospital and Community Psychiatry* 1988; 39: 963–6.

18. Sullivan G, Wells KB, Morgenstern H, Leake B. Identifying modifiable risk factors for rehospitalization: a case-control study of seriously mentally ill persons in Mississippi. *American Journal of Psychiatry* 1995; 152: 1749–56.

19. Akerblad A-C, Finn Bengtsson F, von Knorringaan L, Ekselius L. Response, remission and relapse in relation to adherence in primary care treatment of depression: a 2-year outcome study. *International Clinical Psychopharmacology* 2006; 21: 117–24.

20. Sirey J, Bruce M, Alexopoulos GS, Perlick DA, Raue P, Friedman SJ, Meyers BS. Perceived stigma as a predictor of treatment discontinuation in young and older outpatients with depression. *American Journal of Psychiatry* 2001; 158: 479–81.

21. Sirey J, Bruce M, Alexopoulos GS, Perlick DA, Friedman SJ, Meyers BS. Stigma as a barrier to recovery: perceived stigma and patient-rated severity of illness as predictors of antidepressant drug adherence. *Psychiatric Services* 2001; 52: 1615–20.

22. Paykel Es, Hart D, Priest R. Changes in public attitudes to depression during the defeat depression campaign. *British Journal of Psychiatry* 1998; 173: 519–22.

23. Jorm AF, Christensen H, Griffiths KM. Belief in the harmfulness of antidepressants: Results from a national survey of the Australian public. *Journal of Affective Disorders* 2005; 88(1): 47–53.

24. Althaus D, Stefanek J, Hasford J, Hegerl U. Knowledge and attitudes of the general population towards symptoms, causes, and treatment of depressive disorders. *Der Nervenarzt* 2002; 73(7): 659–64.

25. van Schaik DJF, Klijn AFJ, van Hout HP, van Marwijk HW, Beekman AT, de Haan M, van Dyck R. Patients' preferences in the treatment of depressive disorder in primary care. *General Hospital Psychiatry* 2004; 26(3): 184–9.

26. Col N, Fanale Je, Kronholm P. The role of medication noncompliance and drug reactions in hospitalizations of the elderly. *Archives of Internal Medicine* 1990; 150: 841–5.

27. Gonzalez J, Williams JW, Noel PH, Lee S. Adherence to mental health treatment in a primary care clinic. *Journal of the American Board of Family Practice* 2005; 18(2): 87–96.

28. Aikens JE, Kroenke K, Swindle RW, Eckert GJ. Nine-month predictors and outcomes of SSRI antidepressant continuation in primary care. *General Hospital Psychiatry* 2005; 27(4): 229–36.

29. Linden M, Gothe H, Dittman R, Schaff B. Early termination of antidepressant drug treatment. *Journal of Clinical Psychopharmacology* 2000; 20(5): 523–30.

30. Ashton Ak, Jamerson Bd, Weinstein Wl, Wagoner C. Antidepressant-related adverse effects impacting treatment compliance: results of a patient survey. *Current Therapeutic Research* 2005; 66(2): 96–106.

31. Maddox JC Levi M, Thompson C. The compliance with antidepressants in general practice. *Journal of Psychopharmacology* 1994; 8: 48–53.

32. Demyttenaere K, Enzlin KP, Dewé W, Boulanger B, De Bie J, De Troyer W, Mesters P. Compliance with antidepressants in a primary care setting. 1: Beyond lack of efficacy and adverse events. *Journal of Clinical Psychiatry* 2001; 62(Suppl 22): 30–3.

33. Ayalon L, Arean PA, Alvidrez J. Adherence to antidepressant medications in black and Latino elderly patients. *American Journal of Geriatric Psychiatry* 2005; 13(7): 572–80.
34. Bull SA, Hu XH, Hunkeler EM, Lee JY, Ming EE, Markson LE, Fireman B. Discontinuation of use and switching of antidepressants – influence of patient–physician communication. *Journal of the American Medical Association* 2002; 288(11): 1403–1409.
35. Bulloch AG, Adair CE, Patten SB. Forgetfulness: a role in noncompliance with antidepressant treatment. *Canadian Journal of Psychiatry* 2006; 51(11): 719–22.
36. Maddigan SL, Farris KB, Keating N, Wiens CA, Johnson JA. Predictors of older adults' capacity for medication management in a self-medication program: a retrospective chart review. *Journal of Aging and Health* 2003; 15(2): 332–52.
37. Hansen DG, Vach W, Rosholm J-U, Søndergaard J, Gram LF, Kragstrup J. Early discontinuation of antidepressants in general practice: association with patient and prescriber characteristics. *Family Practice* 2004; 21: 623–9.
38. Montgomery SA, Henry J, McDonald G, Dinan T, Lader M, Hindmarch I, Clare A, Nutt D. Selective serotonin reuptake inhibitors: meta-analysis of discontinuation rates. *International Clinical Psychopharmacology* 1994; 9: 47–53.
39. Anderson IM, Tomenson BM. Treatment discontinuation with selective serotonin reuptake inhibitors compared with tricyclic antidepressants: a meta-analysis. *British Medical Journal* 1995; 310: 1433–8.
40. Barbui C, Hotopf M, Freemantle N, Boynton J, Churchill R, Eccles MP, Geddes JR, Hardy R, Lewis G, Mason JM. Selective serotonin reuptake inhibitors versus tricyclic and heterocyclic antidepressants: comparison of drug adherence. *Cochrane Database of Systematic Reviews* 2000; (4): CD002791.
41. Keene MS, Eaddy MT, Mauch RP, Regan TS, Shah M, Chiao E. Differences in compliance patterns across the selective serotonin reuptake inhibitors. *Current Medical Research Opinion* 2005; 21: 1651–8.
42. van Dulmen S, Sluijs E, van Dijk L, de Ridder D, Heerdink R, Bensing J. Patient adherence to medical treatment: a review of reviews. *BMC Health Services Research* 2007; 7: 55.
43. Guthrie RM. The effects of postal and telephone reminders on compliance with pravastatin therapy in a national registry: results of the first myocardial infarction risk reduction program. *Clinical Therapeutics* 2001; 23: 970–80.
44. Bower P, Gilbody S, Richards D, Fletcher J, Sutton A. Collaborative care for depression in primary care – making sense of a complex intervention: systematic review and meta-regression. *British Journal of Psychiatry* 2006; 189: 484–93.
45. Williams JW, Gerrity M, Holsinger T, Dobscha S, Gaynes B, Dietrich A. Systematic review of multifaceted interventions to improve depression care. *General Hospital Psychiatry* 2007; 29(2): 91–116.
46. Bower P, Gilbody S, Richards D, Fletcher J, Sutton A. Collaborative care for depression in primary care: Making sense of a complex intervention: systematic review and meta-regression. *British Journal of Psychiatry* 2006; 189: 484–93.
47. Pampallona S, Bollini P, Tibaldi G, Kupelnick B, Munizza C. Patient adherence in the treatment of depression. *British Journal of Psychiatry* 2002; 180: 104–109.

48. Peterson A, Takiya L, Finley R. Meta-analysis of trials of interventions to improve medication adherence. *American Journal of Health-System Pharmacy* 2003; 60: 657–65.
49. Bollini P, Pampallona S, Kupelnick B, Tibaldi G, Munizza C. Improving compliance in depression: a systematic review of narrative reviews. *Journal of Clinical Pharmacy and Therapeutics* 2006; 31(3): 253–60.
50. Vergouwen AC, Bakker A, Katon WJ, Verheij TJ, Koerselman F. Improving adherence to antidepressants: a systematic review of interventions. *Journal of Clinical Psychiatry* 2003; 64(12): 1415–20.
51. Myers ED, Calvert EJ. The effect of forewarning on the occurrence of side-effects and discontinuance of medication in patients on amitriptyline. *British Journal of Psychiatry* 1973; 122: 461–4.
52. Myers ED, Calvert EJ. The effect of forewarning on the occurrence of side-effects and discontinuance of medication in patients on dothiepin. *Journal of International Medical Research* 1976; 4: 237–40.
53. Myers ED, Calvert EJ. Information, compliance and side-effects: a study of patients on antidepressant medication. *British Journal of Clinical Pharmacology* 1984; 17: 21–25.
54. Myers ED, Calvert EJ. Knowledge of side effects and perseverance with medication. *British Journal of Psychiatry* 1978; 132: 526–7.
55. Altamura AC, Mauri M. Plasma concentrations, information and therapy adherence during long-term treatment with antidepressants. *British Journal of Clinical Pharmacology* 1985; 20: 714–16.
56. Desplenter FAM, Franciska AM, Simoens S, Laekeman G. The impact of informing psychiatric patients about their medication: a systematic review. *Pharmacy World and Science* 2006; 28(6): 329–41.
57. Myers ED, Branthwaite A. Out-patient compliance with antidepressant medication. *British Journal of Psychiatry* 1992; 160: 83–6.
58. Peveler R, George C, Kinmonth AL, Campbell M, Thompson C. Effect of antidepressant drug counselling and information leaflets on adherence to drug treatment in primary care: randomised controlled trial. *BMJ* 1999; 319: 612–15.
59. Mundt JC, Clarke GN, Burroughs D, Brenneman DO, Griest JH. Effectiveness of antidepressant pharmacotherapy: The impact of medication compliance and patient education. *Depression and Anxiety* 2001; 13: 1–10.
60. Atherton-Naj A, Hamilton R, Riddle W, Naji S. Improving adherence to antidepressant drug treatment in primary care: a feasibility study for a randomized controlled trial of educational intervention. *Primary Care Psychiatry* 2001; 7: 61–7.
61. Akerblad, A-C, Bengtsson F, Ekselius L, Von Knorring, LA. Effects of an educational compliance enhancement programme and therapeutic drug monitoring on treatment adherence in depressed patients managed by general practitioners. *International Clinical Psychopharmacology* 2003; 18(6): 347–54.
62. Bull SA, Hunkeler EM, Lee JY et al. Discontinuing or switching selective serotonin-reuptake inhibitors. *Annals of Pharmacotherapy* 2002; 36(4): 578–84.
63. Garfield S, Francis SA, Smith FJ. Building concordant relationships with patients starting antidepressant medication. *Patient Education and Counseling* 2004; 55(2): 241–6.

64. Arora NK, McHorney CA. Patient preferences for medical decision making – who really wants to participate? *Medical Care* 2000; 38(3): 335–41.
65. Maidment R, Livingston G, Katona C. 'Just keep taking the tablets': adherence to antidepressant treatment in older people in primary care. *International Journal of Geriatric Psychiatry* 2002; 17(8): 752–7.
66. Sleath B, Rubin RH, Huston SA. Hispanic ethnicity, physician-patient communication, and antidepressant adherence. *Comprehensive Psychiatry* 2003; 44(3): 198–204.
67. Young HN, Bell RA, Epstein RM, Feldman MD Kravitz RL. Types of information physicians provide when prescribing antidepressants. *Journal of General Internal Medicine* 2006; 21(11): 1172–7.
68. Stevenson FA, Cox K, Britten N, Dundar Y. A systematic review of the research on communication between patients and health care professionals about medicines: the consequences for concordance. *Health Expectations* 2004; 7: 235–45.
69. Lin EH, Von Korff M, Katon W et al. The role of the primary care physician in patients' adherence to antidepressant therapy. *Medical Care* 1995; 33(1): 67–74.
70. Brown C, Battista DR, Sereika SM, Bruehlman RD, Dunbar-Jacob J, Thase ME. How can you improve antidepressant adherence? Talk to your patients about side effects and how long treatment will take. *Journal of Family Practice* 2007; 56(5): 356–63.
71. Aikens JE, Nease Jr DE, Nau DP, Klinkman MS, Schwenk TL. Adherence to maintenance-phase antidepressant medication as a function of patient beliefs about medication. *Annals of Family Medicine* 2005; 3(1): 23–30.
72. Mitchell AJ. Adherence behaviour with psychotropic medication is a form of self-medication. *Medical Hypotheses* 2007; 68(1): 12–21.

13

Borderline Personality Disorder: Causal Factors, Diagnosis and Treatment

Daniel C. Riordan and Pat Hughes

Ms K was a 32-year-old primary school teacher who sought psycho-therapy for recurrent depression. She was currently employed, having lost several jobs previously because of friction with colleagues. In her present job she was highly critical of her immediate manager, and was on probation in her employment because she had taken so much time off from work. She reported severe stress related to angry confrontation with other staff. She had had several sexual relationships with men, which seemed to have broken down because of her increasing demands for their attention, and her feeling that they pushed her away when she was emotionally distressed. She had been treated intermittently for depression with antidepressants by her general practitioner throughout her adult life, and twice in the previous 5 years had been seen in an emergency department following an overdose of prescribed medication.

Stern introduced the term 'borderline personality' in 1938, with the condition conceived as being on the boundary between neurosis and psychosis, with features of both. Over the subsequent 40 years, clinicians continued to recognise a group of disturbed individuals who were neither psychotic nor neurotic, but who were peculiarly difficult to treat, with high levels of affective distress, chaotic relationships, and having a striking capacity to sabotage their treatment and to create intense frustration in those who attempted to help them. This is well illustrated in Main's classic paper 'The ailment',[1] which vividly describes the disruptive impact these patients may have on individual staff and teams within health services. In addition, these patients use healthcare services more frequently than any other psychiatric group.[2]

The medical and social costs of this prevalent condition are considerable, with recent estimates of the cost per patient estimated to be almost 17,000 euros per year, of which only 22% is for health care.[3]

Nosology and diagnosis

The nosological status of borderline personality disorder (BPD), as distinct from the broader notion of borderline personality, was first established in 1979, with Spitzer and colleagues' description of 'a constellation of relatively enduring personality features of instability and vulnerability with important treatment and outcome correlates'.[4] The following year, and using Spitzer's criteria, the American Psychiatric Association included the category of BPD for the first time in the *Diagnostic and Statistical Manual of Mental Disorders* (DSM-III). BPD is classified on 'Axis II', as an underlying personality condition, rather than 'Axis I' for more circumscribed mental disorders. The category remained in DSM-III-R (1987) and in DSM-IV (1994), with some modifications, but maintaining most of the core symptoms originally outlined.

The DSM-IV diagnosis of BPD requires any five out of nine criteria to be present for a significant period of time. These are:

1. frantic efforts to avoid abandonment
2. a pattern of unstable and intense relationships
3. identity disturbance; unstable self-image
4. impulsivity
5. suicidal and self-harming behaviour
6. affective instability; highly reactive mood
7. chronic sense of emptiness
8. inappropriate intense anger
9. transient paranoid ideation.

In parallel with the appearance of the diagnosis in DSM-III, the *International Classification of Diseases* (ICD-9) included the category of BPD (301.83) in 1977. By 1992, the ICD-10 classification had been further refined, with the category of Emotionally Unstable Personality Disorder (F60.3) being subdivided into Impulsive Type (F60.30) and Borderline Type (F60.31).

The ICD-10 diagnosis of BPD requires evidence of general personality malfunction, where the individual's characteristic patterns of inner experience and behaviour deviate markedly from the culturally expected and accepted range (norm), manifest in cognition, affectivity, impulse control and handling of interpersonal situations. In addition, the individual must show at least three of the following:

1. tendency to act without considering the consequences
2. tendency to conflicts, especially when criticised
3. liability to outbursts of anger
4. difficulty in maintaining action that does not offer immediate reward
5. unstable mood

and at least two of the following:

1. uncertain self-image
2. intense and unstable relationships
3. fear of abandonment
4. threats of self-harm
5. chronic sense of emptiness.

Patients with a diagnosis of BPD frequently show symptoms outside the core diagnostic group, leading to concomitant diagnoses. Comorbid conditions may include serious depressive episodes, eating disorders, anxiety disorders and substance misuse. Post-traumatic stress disorder may be present, most commonly in women who have been sexually abused in childhood.

A substantial proportion of patients with BPD experience serious depression, and one-third to three-quarters self-injure at some time in their lives. Studies of the suicide rate over 10 to 30 years report a range of 3% to 10%. This is around 50 times the rate of the general population.[5] While this is a risk that must be taken seriously, the clinician may at the same time be faced with a patient who attempts to control the therapeutic relationship with threats of self-harm, and management decisions are often taxing for clinical teams.

Aetiology

Developmental studies

A large body of retrospective research has identified associations between BPD and early childhood abuse, trauma and neglect. This work is supported by a prospective study that documented child abuse during subjects' childhood, and found that in young adulthood, child-hood physical abuse, sexual abuse, and neglect were each associated with elevated symptom levels.[6]

Some clinical researchers have argued for extending this environmental aetiological link to encompass a broader range of suboptimal parental care as a cause of BPD, in particular a poor quality of parent–infant attachment.[7] They propose that parental care that does not allow healthy development of affect regulation in the child may lead to subsequent BPD. They point out that the clinging, fearful behaviour, with terror of abandonment, shown by children with a disorganised insecure pattern of attachment is similar to behaviour characteristic of adults with BPD. These children do not expect an appropriate response from a parent when their attachment needs are aroused, and the parent and child show subtle indices of mutually fearful behaviour, even when there is no suspicion of overt abuse. The proposition is that the child fails to receive the repeated contingent response necessary for the normal development of affect regulation.

A number of human studies report associations between childhood abuse or neglect and alterations in brain structure or function. However, this association cannot conclusively show that abuse causes changes in the brain. In support of a causal link, experimental work with animals demonstrates that early abuse or severe stress lead to the subsequent development of epileptiform electroencephalogram (EEG) abnormalities, alterations in the corpus callosum, and reduced volume or synaptic density of the hippocampus.[8]

Genetic vulnerability

Despite the association between neglect and later behavioural disturbance, not all people with BPD have overtly abusive childhood experience, and not all maltreated children develop personality disorder. The question of why some maltreated children appear to be protected from adverse development may relate to genetic factors. A functional polymorphism in the gene occurring in the neurotransmitter-metabolising enzyme monoamine oxidase A (MAO_A) moderates the effect of maltreatment. People who have suffered childhood ill-treatment and whose genetic make-up has led to low MAO_A activity are more likely to engage in antisocial behaviour than abused people with higher MAO_A activity.[9]

An interesting study in monkeys demonstrated that both genetic vulnerability and early experience were necessary for the development of behaviours analogous to BPD. Rhesus monkeys were divided into a group reared by their mothers, and a group separated in early life from the mother and reared with peers. In adult life, only peer-reared monkeys showed impulsive aggressive behaviour, mother-reared monkeys did not. And impulsive aggressive behaviour correlated with lower levels of cerebrospinal fluid (CSF) 5-hydroxyindoleacetic acid (5-HIAA), which did not occur among monkeys reared by their mothers. Within the peer-reared group, it was found that low CSF 5-HIAA depended on the presence of the serotonin-transporter gene (*5-HTT*). Thus, impulsive aggression depended in part on the presence of the gene, and in part on early experience.[10]

Pathology

Neuropathology

Magnetic resonance imaging (MRI) studies of people diagnosed with BPD have shown reduced brain volumes in the amygdala and limbic systems. Positron emission tomography (PET) scans reveal hypometabolism of glucose in the prefrontal cortex and limbic systems. This may be interpreted as showing that, in people with BPD, the 'rational' prefrontal cortex fails to regulate the 'impulsive' limbic system. To use the analogy of a horse and rider, affective brain structures (the horse) run out of control, while the cognitive areas (the rider) lack the strength, experience or skill to rein in this excess activity.[11]

Psychopathology

The two most important factors generally agreed to underlie the symptoms of BPD include *impulsive aggression*, which relates to the more disruptive symptoms of BPD, including poor impulse control, self-mutilation, suicidality and other violent behaviours; and *affect dysregulation* which relates to depression, a sense of emptiness and to poor interpersonal functioning. Other features include aggressiveness as a primary temperamental feature, or secondary to severe abuse; an impaired sense of autonomy, leading to inability to tolerate being alone; and a poor sense of self/identity.

Fonagy and Bateman offer a coherent model of psychopathology based on attachment.[7] They propose that in healthy development the child acquires the ability to represent emotions from having repeated experiences of his own emotional state being accurately recognised. Repeated, consistent experience of this recognition allows the infant to establish a sense of confidence about his mental state, and eventually a mental representation of, and ability to recognise, his own affect. He achieves a sense of being connected with others and being able to communicate his feelings. The parent's inability to do this is liable to lead to the child's internalising the caregiver, with the establishment of an alien identity, rather than his own. Further, it is important that the parent is able to deal with a highly aroused infant, and can calm him when he is distressed. The infant's repeated experience of high arousal followed by calming ultimately leads to an established pattern, which we may assume is represented in the frontal cortex, and leads to appropriate affect regulation. The healthy adult is able to calm himself when upset, unlike the person with BPD, for whom high arousal is hard to alleviate, and who may resort to maladaptive strategies (cutting, binge eating, etc.) to self-calm.

A traumatised child may, in adult life, respond to perceived threat by identifying with the aggressor, or the internalised abusing parent, leading to intense feelings of internal attack, and an overwhelming sense of 'badness'. In an attempt to cope, the individual may dissociate, and show fragmentation of his mental state.

Psychological defence mechanisms commonly shown by patients with BPD

Patients with BPD commonly use so-called 'primitive' defence mechanisms, which are characteristic of the way in which a small child normally relates to the world. These patients, like children, tend to see the world as black and white, all bad or all good. This is especially the case in relation to situations where there is an emotional attachment, especially where the relationship is more intimate. In such relationships, the individual is sensitive to real or imagined slights or disappointments. The defence mechanisms adopted include:

1. splitting
2. projective identification.

Within the mind, aspects of the self with other important individuals are represented. At a simple level, and very notably in BPD patients, this will include a completely satisfied self with a gratifying parent, and a deeply frustrated self with a depriving parent. In times of stress, for example when the individual with BPD is unexpectedly disappointed, they become highly anxious, feel deprived and persecuted, and immediately split the depriving parent image from the mental representation, and project it onto the person, therapist, or service that is perceived as failing him. They then enact the mental model with that person, usually becoming both very upset and very angry. This underlies the attacking behaviour that is very characteristic of patients with BPD when they are in the care of healthcare professionals.

The individual with BPD is also capable of identifying another person as ideal, entirely loving and gratifying, and may be unable to perceive that person as less than perfect. While this may be pleasant for a time, it has a tendency to be precarious: as soon as the idealised other disappoints, they are liable to be perceived as entirely bad and to be denigrated furiously.

Epidemiology and course

BPD is estimated to occur in 10–20 per cent of the psychiatric population.[12] A review of eight epidemiological studies reported the mean prevalence in the general population to be 1.16%.[13]

Until recently it was believed that BPD followed a chronic and largely unremitting course, but recent research suggests that a substantial proportion of individuals are likely to improve significantly over 6 to 10 years. Many will not be free of symptoms, but the disorder may become much less troublesome with time. Two recent prospective studies offer impressive data indicating that the majority of BPD patients show improvement.[14,15] These researchers reported that among patients whose BPD was severe enough to warrant hospital admission, 50% had achieved remission using standard DSM diagnostic criteria 4 years later, and 75% had remitted 6 years later.

However, it was notable that the symptom reduction was behavioural: self-harm, suicidality and impulsivity were much improved, while interpersonal difficulties and affective symptoms were largely unchanged. Substance misuse was related to poorer outcome, suggesting that early intervention targeting this problem is important.

Bateman and Fonagy argue that the gloomy prognosis previously expected may relate to inappropriate treatment interventions.[16] They point out that while it is easily accepted that pharmacological treatments may harm as well as help, it has been too easily assumed that psychological interventions are harmless at worst. If such treatments are seen as a force that can affect mental processes, they may also have a potentially adverse impact on vulnerable individuals, for example by overstimulating rather than containing or calming people whose affect control is already precarious.

Treatment

Treatment of people with BPD has lagged behind the diagnosis of the condition for a two reasons:

1. a lack of effective treatments and research into the effectiveness of these

2. these patients often engender frustration, chaotic thinking, and consequent rejection in health professionals.

Evidence-based treatment of BPD

There is an increasing body of data showing the effectiveness of certain treatments, and the evidence base is growing. Problems that complicate research include:

1. patients with BPD are not a homogenous group and the diagnostic criteria allow for a substantial range and severity of symptoms
2. patients with BPD have longstanding and complex symptoms, and the effectiveness of quick solutions is likely to be short lived. Thus, research has to continue evaluation many months after treatment is completed
3. patients' symptoms can alter on a moment-by-moment basis, so evaluating whether a symptom is made worse or better overall can be difficult
4. confounding factors include comorbid conditions, patient preference and therapist experience and training.

Available evidence suggests that structured psychological treatment is better than non-structured although it is unclear what mechanism allows therapeutic change to take place. In addition, American Psychiatric Association guidelines recommend targeted pharmacotherapy with psychotherapy.

Psychopharmacological treatment

While treatment of BPD depends primarily on psychological interventions, short-term drug treatment may offer symptom relief, and is included in the American Psychiatric Association recommendations of 2001 for treatment of BPD. Both low-dose atypical antipsychotics and selective serotonin reuptake inhibitors (SSRIs) may improve regulation of affect, impulse control and anxiety, and may allow the patient to use psychological treatments more effectively.[17]

Psychological treatments

Several treatment approaches have been evaluated and are shown to offer significant improvement. The features that they share are:

1. a structured approach
2. a coherent theory to underpin the treatment

3. they are long term rather than short term, characteristically lasting 1–3 years

4. a treatment that is organised to contain and survive the patient's attacks on its effective delivery.

Psychological treatments demonstrated to be effective for people with BPD include:

1. dialectical behaviour therapy
2. schema-focused therapy
3. transference-focused therapy
4. mentalisation-based therapy.

Other treatment approaches that have a lesser evidence base but have shown improvement for patients with BPD include cognitive analytic therapy,[18] and treatment within a residential therapeutic community.[19]

Dialectical behaviour therapy

Dialectical behaviour therapy (DBT) was the first treatment that specifically addressed the problems of people with BPD and that showed that this systematic approach could help these difficult and distressed patients. DBT was developed in the 1990s by Marsha Linehan, whose randomised controlled trials demonstrated that DBT was significantly superior to treatment as usual.[20] DBT is manualised and therapists stick as closely as possible to the recommended structure. Therapy for BPD is generally offered as 3–3.5 hours per week for one year.

The treatment is based on cognitive and behavioural methods, with spiritual ideas from Zen Buddhism. The theory underpinning DBT is that an emotionally vulnerable person grows up in an 'invalidating environment' – one where the child's responses are disqualified and rendered maladaptive. The child is not helped to cope with the overwhelming feelings he experiences. 'Dialectic' describes a particular form of reasoning in classical philosophy. Instead of swinging between two poles, a synthesis of opposing notions exist; such that 'either/or' thinking is replaced by 'both/and', to enable a shared understanding between therapist and patient. The relationship between the therapist and patient is central, and staff support is an integral part of the therapy.

Therapy takes place in four arenas: individual, group, telephone and therapist consultation. Treatment focuses on a formulation of the patient's difficulties and a behavioural analysis of his self-harm/suicidal behaviour. The patient makes a commitment to reduce parasuicidal behaviour, address 'therapy-interfering behaviours' and reduce behaviours that interfere with his quality of life. Skills training includes some ideas from Zen Buddhism, such as mindfulness training, which encourages individuals to live in the moment and feel appropriately in charge of the self. The encouragement of other skills includes how to deal with relationships and emotions, and how to develop strategies to manage high levels of distress.

The therapist allows out-of-session telephone contact. This is not an alternative to the therapy session, but is to encourage engagement, avoid self-harm, and repair the therapeutic relationship before the next therapy session. Available times are negotiated, but if they are misused this will be seen as 'therapy-interfering behaviour' and the contract will be renegotiated.

While the therapist treats the patient with DBT, he is supported by colleagues who 'treat' him with the same dialectical techniques. This supportive structure allows the therapist to continue to work with very demanding patients.

Schema-focused therapy

Schema-focused therapy (SFT) derives from cognitive-behavioural therapy (CBT) with a psychodynamic influence. It was developed by Jeffrey Young, who explains that problems in patients with BPD stem from deep-rooted psychological problems constructed as 'schemas' – repetitive life patterns and themes.[21] Patients are warned that patterns of behaviour that become established are familiar and comfortable, and are likely to resist change, even when they are maladaptive. In the treatment of BPD, weekly treatment for 3 years has been shown to be effective.[22]

The therapist identifies 'life traps' that relate to early experience and that continue to be used in a way that impacts adversely on the patient's life. Examples include having an overprotective parent, which may lead to dependency, or having an overindulgent parent may engender an unhelpful sense of entitlement in the child. Both of these scenarios will cause problems if they persist into adult life.

The next step is to explain to the patient that we are drawn to others who will play a role in the established and familiar relationships. Thus, a dependent person will be attracted to a partner who encourages dependency.

The therapist also assures the patient that he has a healthy part to his personality, and encourages a dialogue between the disabled and the healthy aspects of the patient, where maladaptive schema are challenged and alternatives sought. Change is achieved through a range of behavioural, cognitive and experiential techniques that focus on (1) the therapeutic relationship, (2) daily life outside therapy, and (3) past traumatic experiences. Intervention also includes analysis of the trans-ference relationship, with a specific focus on the here and now.

Transference-focused psychotherapy

Transference-focused psychotherapy (TFP) is based on psychoanalytic/psychodynamic concepts.[23] It is a manualised treatment, usually offered twice weekly for up to 3 years. TFP emphasises the importance of the assessment and on establishing a treatment contract that gives a con-taining structure aimed at reducing destructive behaviours during the treatment. The patient is treated as an equal collaborator in agreeing this contract.

The theoretical understanding of BPD psychopathology in TFP is that the mind is split into non-integrated parts, with a tendency for the self and others to be perceived as entirely good or bad. It includes an object relations model where relationships are represented as either idealised and highly gratifying, or frustrating and highly distressing. The patient's tendency to oscillate between these two extremes is dem-onstrated in the emotional swings and chaotic interpersonal relations that he experiences.

Therapy uses interpretation of the transference relationship where these extremes are enacted, and is directed towards helping the indi-vidual to integrate the extremes into a more realistic experience of relationships that have both good and bad components. Importantly, the therapist also helps the patient identify and tolerate the intense affective states that accompany his relationships. The therapist actively interprets unconscious wishes and fears. The aim of treatment is to help the patient modify the extreme states that he is subject to, to integrate fragmented states, and thus to better manage his personal and work life.

Mentalisation-based therapy

Mentalisation-based therapy (MBT) combines some of the techniques of cognitive psychology, along with psychodynamic principles relating to attachment theory. In contrast to TFP, MBT does not use transfer-ence interpretations, nor does the therapist make many interpretations of unconscious motives. The theoretical basis for the approach derives largely from understanding the development of BPD as a failure in healthy attachment (see earlier), and thus an impairment of the patient's ability to accurately represent his own and others' mental state. The therapist actively uses his own mentalising to help the patient learn to mentalise for himself or herself.[24,25]

The key features of the approach are:

1. an exclusive focus on the patient's current mental state (thoughts, feelings, wishes) to help him build accurate representations of mental states
2. avoiding talking about situations where the patient cannot link the mental state to reality. Thus the focus is on conscious or near-conscious content, rather than unconscious, and there is less focus on the past and more on the present
3. the aim is not insight (as in traditional psychoanalytic treatment) but achievement of mentalisation, with an ability to coherently represent the patient's own and others' integrated mental states
4. the therapist makes 'small interpretations' that very slightly push the boundary of the patient's conscious thinking. The therapist avoids complex interpretation of conflict, ambivalence or unconscious motives
5. thus the therapist aims to create a transitional area of relatedness where thoughts and feelings can be 'played with'
6. enactments during treatment are not subjected to interpretation of unconscious motives, but the focus is on the feelings and situations that were immediately associated with them, or acted as triggers.

Treatment outside a specialist setting

Clinicians' attitudes are likely to be more positive for a condition that has a more optimistic prognosis than previously believed. However, untreated, symptom improvement in BPD tends to be in the more external problems: suicidality, self-harm and quasi-psychotic thinking, while symptoms like emptiness, fear of abandonment and depression are more likely to persist, at great cost to the individual.[16] It is therefore important to seek to provide appropriate treatments for these symptoms, and to ensure that clinicians are aware that effective treatment is possible. Regrettably, appropriate specific treatments and services are not currently available at the level required for many people who suffer from this distressing condition. Inevitably, community mental health teams, primary care services, and other agencies will continue to provide clinical care for patients with BPD.

As a group, patients with BPD are often difficult to manage, especially when they are treated outside an experienced specialist service. They often present in crisis after an episode of self-harm, will have difficulty in being reliable in cooperating with treatment, and subject clinical staff to confusing experiences of idealisation or denigration, often within a very short time. Their capacity to divide a team by idealising some members and denigrating others is striking. Teams outside specialist psychotherapy services may usefully take account of the principles of the most effective therapies: agreeing a care plan with the patient, offering structure and problem solving rather than interpretation, ensuring consistency in clinical care with as few changes in key therapeutic staff as possible, working together in the team to avoid splits, and accepting that management will be a long-term commitment.

Conclusions

People with personality disorder occupy an ambivalent place in the hearts of psychiatric professionals, and the debate continues about the rightful setting for the care or disposal of difficult-to-treat patients whose symptoms may appear to be largely self-generated as their injuries are self-inflicted. Where resources are limited, it is often argued that they should not be seen within healthcare services, resulting in the more severely disturbed and disruptive patients ending up in within the prison service. Others remain as 'difficult' people in the community, dealt with, if at all, by general practice or counselling services.

Negative attitudes towards people with personality disorder are now challenged by the increasing body of research demonstrating the aetiological roots of BPD, its neuropathology and psychopathology, and, crucially, the effectiveness of treatments. However challenging the patients, they suffer greatly, and it is the responsibility of the health professions to champion their right to treatment, and to insist that health service managers and politicians recognise and respond to the need for this to be provided.

Key learning points

- Borderline personality disorder (BPD) is a common condition, occurring in over 1% of the general population.
- There is a high rate of associated comorbidity, especially with affective disorders, substance abuse and eating disorders. In addition, more than half of people with the disorder harm themselves, and the suicide rate is 50 times that of the general population.

● Early adverse experience has long been recognised as an aetiological factor; more recently genetic vulnerability has also been implicated.
● Even without specific treatment, many people with BPD show improvement in behavioural symptoms over time, but affective symptoms and chaotic relationships usually persist unless treated.
● Effective treatments are now available. There is good evidence for the benefit of a package of structured psychotherapy for a year or longer. The addition of low-dose atypical antipsychotics or selective serotonin reuptake inhibitors may improve regulation of affect, impulse control and anxiety, and help the patient use psychological treatments.

Key references

●Bateman A, Fonagy P, editors. *Mentalisation-based Treatment for Borderline Personality Disorder*. A practical guide. Oxford: Oxford University Press; 2006.
●Oldham J. Borderline personality disorder and suicidality. *American Journal of Psychiatry* 2006; 163: 20–6.

References

1. Main T. The ailment. *British Journal of Medical Psychology* 1957; 30(3): 129–45.
2. Bender DS, Dolan RT, Skodol AE, Sanislow CA, Dyck IR, McGlashan TH, Shea MT, Zanarini MC, Oldham JM, Gunderson JG. Treatment utilisation by patients with personality disorders. *American Journal of Psychiatry* 2001; 158(2): 295–302.
3. Van Asselt ADI, Dirksen CD, Arntz A, Severens JL. The cost of borderline personality disorder: societal costs in BPD-patients. *European Psychiatry* 2007; 22(6): 354–61.
4. Spitzer RL, Endicott J, Gibbon M. Crossing the border into borderline personality and borderline schizophrenia: the development of criteria. *Archives of General Psychiatry* 1979; 36: 17–24.
5. Skodol AE, Gunderson JG, Pfohl B, Widiger TA, Livesley WJ, Siever LJ (2002) The borderline diagnosis: 1. Psychopathology, comorbidity and personality and personality structure. *Biological Psychiatry* 2002; 51(12): 936–50.
6. Johnson JG, Cohen P, Brown J, Smailes EM, Bernstein DP. Childhood maltreatment increases risk for personality disorders during early adulthood. *Archives of General Psychiatry* 1999; 56: 600–606.
7. Fonagy P, Bateman AW. Mechanisms of change in mentalisation-based treatment of BPD. *Journal of Clinical Psychology* 2006; 62(4): 411–30.
8. Teicher MH, Tomoda A, Andersen SL. Neurobiological consequences of early stress and childhood maltreatment: are results from human and animal studies comparable? *Annals of the New York Academy of Science* 2006; 1071: 313–323.
9. Capsi A, McClay J, Moffitt TE et al. Role of genotype in the cycle of violence in maltreated children. *Science* 2002; 297: 851–4.

10. Bennett AJ, Lesch KP, Heils A et al. Early experience and serotonin trans-porter gene variation interact to influence primate CNS function. *Molecular Psychiatry* 2002; 7: 118–22.

11. Lis E, Greenfield B, Henry M, Guile JM, Dougherty G. Neuroimaging and genetics of borderline personality disorder: a review. *Journal of Psychiatry and Neuroscience* 2007; 32(3): 162–73.

12. Gunderson JG. *Borderline Personality Disorder: a clinical guide.* Washington DC: American Psychiatric Press; 2001.

13. Torgersen S. (2005). Epidemiology. In: Oldham, JM, skodol AE, Bender DS, editors. *The American Psychiatric Publishing Textbook of Personality Disorders.* Washington, DC: American Psychiatric Publishing, Inc; 2005, p. 129–41.

14. Zanarini MC, Frankenburg FR, Hennen J, Silk KR. The longitudinal course of borderline psychopathology: 6-year prospective follow-up of the phenom-enology of borderline personality disorder. *American Journal of Psychiatry* 2003; 160: 274–83.

15. Shea MT, Stout RL, Yen S et al. Associations in the course of personality dis-orders and axis I disorders over time. *Journal of Abnormal Psychology* 2004; 113: 499–508.

16. Bateman A, Fonagy P. *Mentalization-based Treatment for Borderline Personality Disorder: a practical guide.* Oxford: Oxford University Press; 2006.

17. Soloff P. (2005) Pharmacotherapy in borderline personality disorder. In: Gurderson JG, Hoffman PD, editors. *Understanding and Treating Borderline Personality Disorder.* Washington DC: American Psychiatric Publishing; 2005, p. 65–82.

18. Ryle A, Golynkina K. Effectiveness of time-limited cognitive analytic ther-apy of borderline personality disorder: factors associated with outcome. *British Journal of Medical Psychology* 2000; 73: 197–210.

19. Menzies D, Dolan BM, Norton K. Are short term savings worth long term costs? Funding treatment for personality disorders. *Psychiatric Bulletin* 1993; 17: 517–19.

20. Linehan MM, Armstrong HE, Suarez A, Allmon D, Heard H. Cognitive-behaviour treatment of chronically parasuicidal borderline patients. *Archives of General Psychiatry*, 1991; 48: 1060–4.

21. Young JE. *Cognitive Therapy for Personality Disorders: a schema focused approach.* Sarasota: Professional Resource Press; 1994.

22. Giesen-Bloo J, van Dyck R, Spinhoven P et al. Outpatient psychotherapy for borderline personality disorder: a randomized trial of schema focused therapy versus transference focused therapy. *Archives of General Psychiatry* 2006; 63(6): 649–58.

23. Clarkin JF, Yeomans FE, Kernberg OF. *Psychotherapy for Borderline Personality.* New York: J Wiley and Sons; 1999.

24. Bateman AW, Fonagy P. (1999) The effectiveness of partial hospitalisation in the treatment of borderline personality disorder: a randomised controlled trial. *American Journal of Psychiatry* 1999; 156: 1563–9.

25. Bateman AW, Fonagy P. Treatment of borderline personality disorder with psychoanalytically oriented partial hospitalization: an 18-month follow-up. *American Journal of Psychiatry* 2001; 158: 36–42.

14

Biofeedback in Psychiatric Practice

Kishore Chandiramani

Biofeedback has been defined as a group of therapeutic procedures that utilise external devices (mechanical, electronic or computer) to measure and feedback to the individual information about their physiological functions. These devices can act as a mirror to the mind, and the feedback can help individuals achieve a greater awareness and control over their physiological processes. The external devices may not be required if one is able to establish connections with one's inner state of affairs, as happens in certain types of meditations. In this respect biofeedback can been described as the western equivalent of eastern meditation practices. Keeping their synergistic action in mind, biofeedback and meditation practices have been successfully combined in achieving relief from stress.

With the help of biofeedback devices, it has been possible to change the autonomic nervous system (ANS) functions such as heart rate, peripheral blood flow, skin temperature, brain-wave pattern and smooth muscle activity – which are normally outside voluntary control. Unfortunately, until recently, the use of biofeedback treatment was limited in medicine, and more so in psychiatry. Its lack of popularity in the past could be related to not having very sophisticated equipment that could measure the subtle changes in physiology and convert them into tangible signals. Secondly, within the field of psychiatry, the early research did not show any consistent physiological changes accompanying psychiatric illness, apart from cardiovascular hyperactivity in stress disorders. It is only in recent years that the popularity of this treatment method has grown. Research done in the last decade or so has consistently shown physiological changes in electroencephalograhpy (EEG) patterns, heart-rate variability, etc not just in anxiety disorders but in other psychiatric illnesses as well, giving new hope to psychiatric patients. There now appears to be a distinct role for applied psycho-physiology and biofeedback therapy in the management of psychiatric disorders.

Historical background

Biofeedback therapy was first discovered in the late 1950s in the United States of America (USA) following the realisation that one can change the physiology of one's body by changing the mind. It has its roots in many disciplines such as behaviour therapy, cybernetics, psychophysiology and EEG, consciousness and stress-management strategies.

Early researchers believed that ANS activity or visceral learning could be modified only via classical conditioning, and that even thoughts could become conditioned stimuli and elicit physiological responses. Later studies, done in the 1970s and 1980s showed that operant or instrumental conditioning can also result in changes in ANS functions such as vasomotor responses, blood pressure, salivation, galvanic skin response (GSR) and cardiac rhythm.[1,2]

Claude Bernard, a physician, developed the concept of physiological homoeostasis, which became integral to the discipline of physiology. Illnesses were thought to occur because some homeostatic feedback mechanism was malfunctioning, and a similar homeostatic imbalance was thought to explain stress.[3] The pioneering work done by Cannon and Selye[4] led to the understanding that the physiological stress response and psychosomatic illnesses were results of breakdown in the homeostatic mechanisms. This understanding paved the way for the use of biofeedback therapy in stress disorders.

How does biofeedback work?

At a very simple level, biofeedback seems to work in the same way a mirror works for improving one's physical appearance. Biofeedback has been described as a mirror to the mind or a camera on the unconscious. A simple awareness of something that the person was not conscious of can be therapeutic, as in some instances the individual has got the ability to take remedial measures. For example, after seeing, during an electromyogram (EMG) feedback session, that the tension in his shoulder muscles was 50 microvolts as compared to the normal value of 5 microvolts, a client was able to reduce it by adopting simple relaxation methods.

Psychocybernetics

It is not difficult to understand that the human body has an inbuilt ability to heal itself. This potential for inner healing seems to apply to the mind as well. The efficacy of this natural ability depends upon a number of factors, one of them being the homoeostatic mechanisms. These homeostatic mechanisms work on the principles of cybernetics and are dependent upon an individual's ability to stay connected with the inner feedback signals. From a psychiatric point of view, this would mean staying connected with the inner distress. Biofeedback therapy and meditative practices help clients get in touch with their inner stresses without reacting emotionally to them (or learning to stay relaxed at the same time), hence promoting these homeostatic mechanisms.

Cybernetics is the principle that can explain the self-regulatory function of systems, both animate and inanimate. It is based on the assumption of circular causality, i.e. that the output of a system can be used as an input for the same system in order to modify its function. This principle works for control of room temperature with the help of a thermostat. In living organisms, described as homeostasis, it helps in maintaining blood pressure and blood sugar with the help of baroreceptors and chemoreceptors respectively. Pain control within the body can also be explained on the same principle, i.e. the sensation of pain acts as a feedback signal, which leads to release of endorphins from the brain, resulting in reduction of pain sensation. The same principle applies to the mind as well, and this science has been described as psychocybernetics. It is about providing a feedback to the mind on the physiology or behaviour of an individual, which can lead to regulation or control of the abnormal experience, function or behaviour.

The role of cybernetic principles in biofeedback therapy has been explained in terms of a number of different models, i.e. operant conditioning, homeostasis, information processing,[5] etc. From a cybernetic perspective, operant conditioning is one form of feedback. The individual performs some mental tasks that result in reduction (or increase) in stress scores and this feedback, in the form of positive (or negative) results of a particular behaviour, acts as reinforcer.

Indications for the use of biofeedback therapy

Biofeedback therapy has been successfully used in a number of psychiatric and neurological disorders. Table 14.1 describes some of the examples of the conditions where biofeedback has been used and the

Table 14.1 Disorders and therapeutic modalities used

Disorders	Therapies/modalities
Anxiety and panic disorders	Heart-rate variability training
	Temperature training
Depressive disorders	Heart-rate variability training
Alcohol and drug misuse disorders	Neurofeedback (alpha-theta training)
	Audio-visual entrainment devices
Epilepsy	Neurofeedback
Attention deficit and hyperactivity disorders[6]	Neurofeedback
Psychosomatic disorders such as:	
• tension headaches and migraine[7]	EMG feedback
• irritable bowel syndrome	Heart-rate variability, abdominal breathing
• asthma	Heart-rate variability, abdominal breathing
• hypertension[8]	Paced breathing with the help of E-Z Air™ or respirator
• Raynaud's disease	Temperature training
Urinary and faecal incontinence/ vulvodynia	Surface EMG

Box 14.1 Contraindications of biofeedback therapy

Acute agitation where the client is unlikely to participate in the treatment process
Severe depression with suicidal ideation
Manic disorder
Paranoid states
Severe obsessive-compulsive disorder
Acute medical decompensation
Potential for dissociation, depersonalisation and fugue states

---

therapeutic modality used. Box 14.1 describes contraindications for biofeedback therapy. Box 14.2 outlines the parameters of stress that could be measured as a part of biofeedback therapy.

Important concepts

Heart-rate variability

The rate at which the heart beats varies from beat to beat even in healthy and normal states. In fact, it is considered desirable to have a greater variation in heart beat, as it has been reported that heart-

---

Box 14.2   Parameters of stress that can be measured

Increased muscle tension
Increased respiratory rate
Lowered skin temperature
Increased heart rate (seen during panic attacks)
EEG changes in the alpha, theta, delta and beta waves
Galvanic skin resistance
Peripheral blood flow – indicative of vasoconstriction seen in anxiety disorders

---

rate variability is low in disease states. A measure of variability, usually the standard deviation of the R wave to R wave interbeat interval, is indicative of autonomic control of the heart and perhaps also the lungs, the gut and certain facial muscles.[9] This variability, called heart rate variability (HRV), is controlled by two pathways within the ANS: the sympathetic and parasympathetic. A decreased HRV is associated with increased cardiac mortality and morbidity. Research has discovered a link between respiration rhythm and heart rhythm. A rhythmic braking and speeding of the heart rate is associated with respiration. With inhalation, the vagal (sympathetic) braking is removed, and thus the heart rate is speeded up. The opposite happens during expiration, the vagal brake is reapplied and it slows the rate down again. This heart rate/respiration rhythm is called respiratory sinus arrhythmia (RSA). The finding that heart rate changes with respiration has allowed researchers to modify HRV by way of altering respiratory rhythm. The most commonly used respiratory pattern in biofeedback treatment is abdominal breathing

The role of breathing in biofeedback therapy

Breath can be described as the royal road to the ANS functions. Breathing is one of the very few functions that is voluntary and at the same time autonomous. Breathing slowly (at the rate of five to seven breaths per minute), deeply and into the abdomen (leading to flattening of the diaphragm) has been reported to have a stabilising effect on the heart and gut motility. Different schools of thought recommend different types of breathing as listed next:

● *abdominal breathing* – the practice of abdominal breathing has its roots in yoga and music (opera) traditions. Instead of expanding their upper chest during inspiration, clients learn to push the diaphragm down creating extra space in their chest to breathe in. The individual can see their abdomen rise and fall during respiration while the upper chest remains relatively still. Abdominal breathing has been found to help those who suffer from anxiety, panic attacks, hypertension, irritable bowel syndrome, premenstrual syndromes, sinus tachycardia, etc

- *awareness of breathing (anapana)* – awareness of one's own natural breath is an important first step in the practice of Vipassana meditation.[10] Unlike breath-regulation techniques such as abdominal breathing, it does not involve any conscious effort to change the pattern of one's normal breathing. The individual simply observes the natural flow of his respiration and treats his thoughts and emotions as the background noise. This form of breathing can be seen as a form of biofeedback where the individual becomes aware of the abnormal patterns of breathing such as hyperventilation, breath holding, sighing, etc. A simple awareness of the abnormal pattern can result in resumption of the normal pattern
- *paced breathing* – it has been reported that during the inhalation phase, one's sympathetic nervous system activity is higher compared to the exhalation phase when parasympathetic activity is higher. This principle has been used in modulation of ANS activity. Prolongation of the exhalation phase will therefore result in higher parasympathetic activity, which can be of therapeutic benefit to a client suffering from hypertension and irritable bowel disease. Paced breathing can be learned with the help of software that can be downloaded from the Biofeedback Foundation of Europe website, www.bfe.org. Clients see a dot moving up and down along a graph on the computer screen and try to breathe in when the dot is moving up, and breathe out when the dot is moving down.

The rationale for using biofeedback therapy in psychiatric disorders

Physiological abnormalities have been reported in a number of psychiatric disorders such as anxiety disorders, depressive disorders, alcohol and substance misuse and attention deficit and hyperactivity disorder (ADHD) and in epilepsy.

Anxiety disorders

The activation of sweat glands as part of sympathetic overactivity in anxiety disorders has been known to mental health professionals for some time but the devices initially available were not very accurate and user friendly. The other features of sympathetic overactivity seen in anxiety patients are peripheral vasoconstriction, hyperventilation, increased muscle tone, reduced HRV, etc.

The research on HRV has helped reformulate biological theories of anxiety, shifting the focus of attention away from sympathetic nervous system disturbances in favour of a more balanced approach that considers the interaction between sympathetic and parasympathetic activity. A reduced HRV has been found in several anxiety disorders patients who are found to be at increased risk for coronary heart disease, including sudden death. Individuals with high levels of anxiety have a 4.5- to 6.0-fold increase in risk for sudden cardiac death compared to individuals with no anxiety.[11]

Depressive disorders

Patients suffering from depression have been found to have a right–left asymmetry in the alpha activity on EEG, and this finding has been reported in the offspring of patients suffering from depression who have not had depressive illness.

The right frontal lobe is thought to be involved in the organisation and production of negative emotions and avoidance behaviour. Any damage or deactivation of this part of the brain can result in hypomanic symptoms. The opposite is true for depression, i.e. the left frontal lobe is involved in organisation and production of positive emotions and approach behaviour, and brain insult in this area can cause depression symptoms.[12] Deactivation has been reported to be associated with high alpha activity in that area, which can be modified with the help of neurofeedback therapy.

Neurofeedback therapy

Neurofeedback has been used successfully in ADHD, epilepsy, anxiety disorders, mood disorders, traumatic brain injury and alcohol and substance misuse.[13,14]

There is some evidence to indicate that ADHD patients have reduced beta-wave activity in their brains. Beta waves are commonly associated with cortical arousal. These children, who have under-aroused brains indulge in hyperactive behaviour, in order to bring their cortical arousal to an optimal level. With neurofeedback training, these children can be trained to enhance beta activity, which has therapeutic value. For epilepsy patients, two commonly used protocols are (a) feedback of sensory motor rhythm and (b) based on slow cortical potential.[15]

It has been demonstrated that anxiety disorder patients have fewer alpha waves and more beta waves. This pattern can be altered with the help of EEG feedback. The biofeedback protocols for anxiety disorders include alpha and theta enhancement.[14] Combined alpha–theta EEG feedback procedures have also been used successfully in treating patients with addictive behaviour such as alcoholism.[16–18]

Substance misuse

EEG has been used to measure cortical arousal, which is generally altered in substance-misuse disorders. Individuals who are dependent on alcohol or other central nervous system (CNS) depressants, such as benzodiazepines, opiates, heroin etc, have been reported to have high cortical arousal, with its accompanying high beta and low alpha activity on EEG. They use sedatives in order to bring their cortical arousal to an optimal level. In a similar fashion, individuals who are addicted to the CNS stimulants such as amphetamines and cocaine have been reported to have a lower cortical arousal, with its accompanying low beta activity in their brains. They use stimulants to raise their arousal levels to an optimal level by using stimulants. With neurofeedback, these individuals can be trained to alter their brain-wave patterns, with some therapeutic benefits.

Assessment process

The assessment consists of initial history taking and mental state examination, followed by a psychophysiological assessment. The objective of a psychophysiological assessment is to record the baseline physiological data on EMG, skin conductance, skin temperature and respiratory and cardiac rhythm, followed by a study of the adaptation period following a stress test. The stress test consists of exposing the individual to stress – cognitive (given a complex mathematical task), emotional (asked to imagine a traumatic or stressful experience) or physical (hand in ice-cold water). This exposure results in a physiological stress response, which gradually resolves. The important aspect is to see in how much time the physiological status return to normal levels. The post-stress recovery is more important than the amplitude of change. It has been found that the time period required to recover completely is different for different modalities. For example, for a given individual the skin temperature might take longer to return to normal compared to the heart rate, which returns to normal quickly. The opposite may be true for someone else. Therapists generally work with the modalities that take longer to recover.

Treatment process

Treatment generally begins with educating patients about the rationale for physiological self-regulation, the therapy process, therapy goals, therapy options, lifestyle issues, i.e. diet, work, exercise, leisure, etc. They are encouraged to write a baseline symptom log and are trained in the relaxation method of their choice.

Improvement can start just after one or two sessions but on average clients report satisfactory improvement after about 6 to 12 sessions. Neurofeedback therapy takes a little longer, up to 30 sessions. Each session lasts approximately 30 minutes. The sessions are carried out twice a week initially for a few weeks, followed by less frequent sessions – fortnightly or monthly.

The commonly used treatment approaches for anxiety and panic disorders are HRV training, skin conductance, temperature training and EEG feedback. The HRV training is generally combined with abdominal breathing. The choice of modality depends upon patient responsiveness to stress, and the symptom profile. The EEG feedback that involves alpha/theta enhancement is generally used only when the QEEG demonstrates a decline in alpha activity.

Biofeedback therapy can be combined with any other treatment method with known efficacy, and it is likely to increase the efficacy of those treatment methods by quantifying change and providing feedback in real time. At times, for some patients, a positive change in their scores does not directly translate into symptom relief. The focus of therapy for such patients should shift from just achieving change in the ratings to actual clinical improvement

Biofeedback devices

Multimodal systems

These devices are able to capture data on several modalities simultaneously and can be utilised for a wide variety of applications such as respiration training, HRV, EEG, EMG, ECG, electro-oculography (EOG), skin temperature, blood volume pulse, skin conductance, oximetry, capnography, etc. The sensors for these modalities can be combined in many different configurations. The two commercially available devices are NEXUS-10[19] and BioGraph Infiniti.[20] Nexus is a 10-channel physiological monitoring and feedback platform that utilises Blue Tooth technology for wireless recording of data.

Unimodal systems

Emwave

• Emwave is a portable device that has been used to lower stress levels by way of increasing heart-rhythm coherence. Coherence is a term used to describe a state of harmony between the heart, respiration and nervous system. It measures the variation in heart rate and also the pattern that variation follows in relation to the respiration pattern, in order to calculate the coherence scores. The scores are depicted as low, medium and high and the feedback is provided in terms of different-coloured lights, indicating different levels of coherence, i.e. red for low, blue for medium and green for high. The goal is to reduce stress by achieving and sustaining high coherence (green light).[21]

The Journey to Wild Divine

• This measures skin conductance levels and heart rate and has been used to reduce anxiety and stress. The three skin sensors connect through a device called 'stone', an energy translator that converts signals into computer data that are then converted into multimedia signals. It is very much like playing a video game of adventure on the computer. The individual moves from one stage to the next, only when they have mastered the tasks given to them during this interactive game, through practice of relaxation and breathing exercises. *www.wilddivine.com*

Resperate

• Resperate is a battery-operated, hand-held device that analyses the breath pattern first and then gradually guides the individual to change it, i.e. reduce breathing rate and prolong exhalation. It reduces the neural sympathetic activity and relaxes the small blood vessels. Resperate has been shown to reduce high blood pressure. It utilises the principle of paced breathing, i.e. prolonging exhalation leads to increased vagal activity, thereby restoring the balance between sympathetic and parasympathetic activity. *www.resperate.co.uk*

Myotrac

• This is a single-channel EMG. Its DC voltage output connects accessories and permits computer monitoring. It has been used for repeti-

tive strain injuries, tension headaches, chronic musculoskeletal pain, pelvic floor muscle training, etc.
www.thoughttechnology.com/myotrac.htm

U-Control

- This is a battery-operated, single-channel, surface EMG training device that is used for muscle re-education in the treatment of urinary and faecal incontinence.[20]
www.futurehealth.org/ucontrol.htm

Skin-conductance devices

- Skin conductance biofeedback has been used for anxiety disorders, peak performance training for athletes, etc (thought stream).
www.affectiva.com

Innovative uses of biofeedback

The potential for altering physiological functions has been used not just to restore homeostasis in disease states but also to increase the levels of performance beyond the normal and to enhance creativity. Biofeedback is increasingly being used for enhancing performance by sportsmen and for improving creativity by musicians, artists, students, etc. Theta waves have been linked with new learning and students have used theta-training protocols on neurofeedback to enhance their memory and other cognitive functions.

In sport medicine, control of muscle tension and emotions and arousal reduction with the biofeedback devices has been found to enhance performance. However, for highly aggressive and combative sports such as football, basketball, hockey, etc, the goals are just the opposite, i.e. intensification of emotional and physical reaction is considered desirable.

Thought-translation devices (TTDs) and language support programmes (LSPs) have enabled paralysed and mute patients to communicate and perform physical tasks, with the help of a direct connection between the brain (EEG) and a computer. Self-regulation of slow cortical potentials is used to control a cursor on the computer screen, which enables the client to perform a number of physical and language tasks. Subjects trained in using TTD have demonstrated playing an orchestra just by changing their brain-wave patterns, and without making any physical movements.

Virtual-reality therapy has been used in recent years, in conjunction with biofeedback devices, in the treatment of anxiety, panic and phobic disorders. It has also been used in combative stress in a military setting for prevention and management of post-traumatic stress disorders.

Conclusions

Biofeedback therapy has provided scientific credibility to a number of treatment approaches such as abdominal breathing, entrainment devices, and other complementary therapies, as one can measure the scores before and after any therapy session to quantify the improvement. It has been successfully combined with a number of different therapies. It is unfortunate that in spite of the scientific evidence supporting the efficacy of biofeedback therapy, its use has remained limited in psychiatric settings. In this respect, psychiatry is lagging behind other disciplines in the use of modern technology.

The evidence supporting the efficacy of biofeedback is growing. Patients like it as they can see for themselves the changes happening as a result of their efforts. They can practise it on their own with very little supervision from the therapist, and as a result feel motivated and empowered.

Key learning points

● Technological advancement has now made it possible to measure accurately the physiological changes associated with psychological stress.
● Several psychological disorders including anxiety and depression are known to be associated with changes in autonomic nervous system functions and heart rate variability, which can be reversed with the help of biofeedback therapy.
● Brain-wave patterns can be modulated with the help of biofeedback devices, resulting in therapeutic benefits for clients suffering from epilepsy, ADHD, substance misuse, etc.

Scientific societies

The following scientific societies promote a greater awareness of biofeedback and, through training workshops, educate clinicians in the use of biofeedback techniques and technology.

● The Association for Applied Psychophysiology and Biofeedback – http://www.aapb.org

- The Biofeedback Foundation of Europe – http://www.bfe.org
- The Society for the Neuronal Regulation – http://www.snr-jnt.org

References

1. Kimmel HO. Instrumental conditioning of autonomically mediated responses in human beings. *American Psychologist* 1979; 29: 325–35.
2. Harris AH, Brady JV. Animal learning: visceral and autonomic conditioning. *Annual Review of Psychology* 1974; 25: 107–33.
3. Schwartz MS, Olson RP. Historical perspective on the field of biofeedback and applied psychophysiology. In: Schwartz M, Andrasik F, editors. *Biofeedback: a Practitioner's Guide.* London: Guilford Press; 2003, 3–19.
4. Cannon WB. Organization for physiological homeostasis. *Physiol Rev* July 1929; 9(3): 399–431.
   Selye H. *The stress of life.* New York, NY, US: McGraw-Hill; 1956; xvi, 324.
5. Anliker J. Biofeedback from the perspective of cybernatics and systems science. In: Beatty J, Legewie H, editors. *Biofeedback and Behaviour.* New York: Plenum Press; 1977, 1–67.
6. Kaiser DA, Othmer S. Effects of neurofeedback on variables of attention in a large multi-centre trial. *Journal of Neurotherapy* 2000; 4: 5–15.
7. Schwartz M, Andrasik F, editors. *Biofeedback: a Practitioner's Guide.* London: Guilford Press; 2003.
8. Yucha CB, Clark L, Smith M Uris P, LAfleur B, Duval S. The effect of biofeedback in hypertension. *Applied Nursing Research* 2001; 14: 29–35.
9. Gevirtz RN, Lehrer P. Resonant frequency heart rate biofeedback. In: Schwartz M, Andrasik F, editors. *Biofeedback: a Practitioner's Guide.* London: Guilford Press; 2003, p. 245–50.
10. Chandiramani K. *Undo your Stress: learn to manage your everyday stress.* www.undoyourstress.com (accessed 4 April 2011).
11. Grillon C. Anxiety disorders: Psychological aspects. In: Sadock BJ and Sadock VA, editors. *Comprehensive Textbook of Psychiatry,* 8th edn. Sadock and Sadock, Philadelphia: Lippincott Williams and Wilkins; 2005, p. 1730.
12. Davidson, RJ. Cerebral asymmetry, emotion, and affective style. In: Davidson RJ, Hugdahl K, editors. *Brain Asymmetry.* Cambridge, MA; MIT Press; 1995, 361–387.
13. Sterman MB, Friar L. Suppression of seizures in epileptics following sensorimotor EEG feedback training. *Electroencephalography and Clinical Neurophysiology* 1972; 33: 89–95.
14. Yucha CB, Gilbert C. *Evidence Based Practice in Biofeedback and Neurofeedback.* Wheat Ridge, CO: AAPB; 2004.
15. Rockstroh B, Elbert T, Canavan AGM, Lutzenberger W, Birmaumer N. *Slow Cortical Potentials and Behaviour,* 2nd edition. Baltimore: Urban and Schwarzenberg; 1989.
16. Orchs L. EEG treatment of addictions. *Biofeedback.* 1992; 20(1): 8–16.
17. Rosenfeld JP. EEG treatment of addictions, commentary on Orchs, Peniston and Kulkosky. *Biofeedback* 1992; 20(2): 12–17.
18. Peniston EC, Kulkosky PJ. Alcoholic personality and alpha-theta brain-wave training. *Medical Psychotherapy* 1990; 3: 37–55.

19. *Mind Media: the Physiological Monitoring and Biofeedback Company.* www.mindmedia.info (accessed 4 April 2011).
20. Thought Technology Ltd. www.thoughttechnology.com (accessed 4 April 2011).
21. HeartMath. http://www.heartmathstore.com/ (accessed 4 April 2011).

Index

Printed in the United States
by Baker & Taylor Publisher Services

Printed in the United States
by Baker & Taylor Publisher Services